# total gut reset

# Total Gut Reset

DR. LAUREN LAX

PIERUCCI
PUBLISHING

Pierucci Publishing books may be purchased in bulk at special discounts for sales promotion, corporate gifts, fund-raising, or educational purposes. Special editions can be created to specifications. For details, contact the Special Sales Department, Pierucci Publishing, PO Box 8067, Aspen, CO 81612.

Publishing@PierucciPublishing.com
Visit our website at www.pieruccipublishing.com.
Hardcover ISBN: 978-1-956257-75-5
Paperback ISBN: 978-1-956257-76-2
Ebook ISBN: 978-1-956257-77-9
Audiobook ISBN: 978-1-956257-78-6
Cover Design by Cortney Walker
Edited by Dale Chaplin
Lauryn's portrait by Juan Valdes
Library of Congress Control Number: 2023902833

# CONTENTS

# DEDICATION

For **mom** and **dad**.
Who taught me what "*gut love*" really means.

And to my mentor **Barbara**.
Who taught me to always go with my gut.

# BOOK DISCLAIMER

This book provides content related to physical and/or health issues. As such, use of this book implies your acceptance of this disclaimer. The information presented is the author's opinion and does not constitute any health or medical advice. The content of this book is for informational purposes only and is not intended to diagnose, treat, cure, or prevent any condition or disease. Understand that this book is not intended as a substitute for consultation with a licensed healthcare practitioner, such as your physician. Before you begin any healthcare program, or change your lifestyle in any way, please seek advice from your licensed healthcare provider for your personal health concerns prior to taking healthcare advice from this book.

# PROLOGUE:
# HEALED TO HEAL OTHERS

***"The best medicine is to teach a person not to need it."***
***-Hippocrates.***

***Today, the philosophy is:***
***"What chemicals can help me heal?" (Including our food system).***

*The problem with society worldwide is that we are all taught from the time we are children to utilize chemicals to treat disease.*

This book is an unconventional book on gut health—why it is important and how to improve it.

Unless you've been living under a rock, you have probably heard that your gut health is pretty important. You've probably heard that it is especially important for your immune system; your gut is where the majority of your immune-fighting cells reside.

However, despite this acknowledgement, there is a lot of conflicting information out there on the topic. In fact, if you're like 80 percent of Americans, you are completely confused and overwhelmed by what the term "healthy" even means, thanks to the five thousand-plus ads you see on a daily basis.

If you're like the majority of Americans who have at least one chronic health condition (from autoimmunity to hypothyroidism, irritable bowel syndrome (IBS), anxiety, allergies, and beyond), you are dealing with "dysbiosis" (a fancy word for a "disrupted microbiota").

Even worse? What you've been told is healthy may not be helping your gut microbiome at all (explaining why 99 percent of all diets fail). This was exactly my case for more than thirty years, and it is what inspired me to write this book so you, too, can learn how to optimize your gut health—especially if you've already been doing all the things you've been told are good for you.

Health is an inside job. Allow me to explain...

## FIBER ONE DOES A BODY GOOD

*1994*

"Mooooomm, my tummy hurts."

Constipated. Constantly. For as long as I could remember, going for a number two was never easy. In response, Mom made an appointment for Dr. Joe to see me and do some scans.

"Well, it looks like she has an enlarged colon, which may explain her chronic constipation. I recommend we increase the fiber and water," Dr. Joe explained. This advice preceded a shift from my old breakfast of Pop-tarts or Cap'n Crunch cereal with a side of banana and Iron Kids bread toast spread with margarine and jelly to a new breakfast of Fiber One cereal with strawberries and whole wheat toast with honey.

This change, however, did not work. I was still constipated.

The Fiber One diet didn't last for long.

## DORITOS

*1996*

"Do you want Doritos or Cheetos?" Mom asked. She was bustling around the kitchen, packing my lunch for school while I sat at the breakfast bar, slurping down the remains of my pink-tinged Lucky Charms milk.

"Duh, Mom!" I said, giggling and pointing to the Doritos. The answer was a no-brainer.

"Okay, great," she said. "Finish up. We need to leave in five minutes." She stuffed the chip bag along with my PB & J on white Iron Kids bread (no crust), grapes, and a Hostess Twinkie (my favorite dessert) into my Strawberry Shortcake lunchbox.

I swigged a final shot of Tropicana orange juice and took one last bite of my mushy banana, still tasting the bubblegum-flavored toothpaste on my recently brushed teeth. Then, I was off to school.

Those were the happy-go-lucky days.

## *DO YOU LIKE ME?* CHECK YES OR NO

*March 1997*

"Psst, Erin, go ask Nate if Eric likes me," I whispered conspiratorially. Fourth Grade recess was where all the juicy stuff happened.

A break from a busy workday spent crunching numbers, memorizing the fifty states, and reading *The Wizard of Oz*. Recess was a time to catch up on the important things, like Samantha's big birthday party, the latest gossip on *N'Sync* and *The Backstreet Boys*, cheerleading stunt contests, and figuring out who liked who for the crush of the moment.

Always a "shy one," I rarely admitted my secret crushes, much less assessed the scene myself to see if that crush liked me back. Nevertheless, I *really* liked Eric Anderson, with his freckled face, Ken-doll gelled hair (minus the cowlick), big goofy ears, a strong chin, and a tall, 4-foot-something stature. In my mind, Eric was the bee's knees. He also happened to be one of the most popular boys in school, destined to be a quarterback or captain of the high school basketball team, had a naturally cool taste in music, and head-turning trendsetter style (hello, Abercrombie & Fitch).

Sure, the other girls liked him, too, but as far as I was concerned, Eric Anderson + me = Happily Ever After.

Finally, I mustered up the guts to have my friend Erin go and ask Eric's sidekick, Nick, if Eric had feelings for me. Waiting patiently on the opposite side of the playground by the swings and gravel, I twisted my feet in the rocks, nervously twirled my hair, and tried not to look their way.

I waited for three minutes, and those three minutes felt like three months of agony. Would we really live happily ever after?

As Erin skipped back to my side, I held my breath and hoped, only to hear:

"No. He's just not that into you... but he *does* like Sarah," Erin said matter-of-factly before scampering away.

I was left with a pit in my stomach, my head down, a lump in my throat, and my heart sinking.

*Not good enough.*

# GOOD ENOUGH

For as long as I can remember, all I ever wanted was to be "good enough." Not necessarily the best, the smartest, or the prettiest, but one of the best, one of the smartest, and one of the prettiest.

Call it being Type A, a child of an upper-middle class pressure cooker, or a tough inner critic, but "good enough" was something I could never seem to attain. Like a carrot dangling in front of a horse's nose, "good enough" kept me striving to take front and center in my annual dance recital and the middle spot at the cafeteria table (where all the popular girls sat). "Good enough" kept me striving to make straight As and land the top of the honor roll, be a "good girl" according to teachers and parents, and be "that girl" who the boys at school liked—dying to talk to me on AOL instant messenger or call my home phone and ask my dad permission to speak to me (when landlines were a thing).

*One day.*

Although I had tons going for me—top student, great dancer, basketball and soccer superstar, lots of friends, an incredible family... in my eyes, "good enough" still didn't exist.

*Health—total health—is an inside job.*

# TUMMY TUCK

Shuffle. Step. Shuffle. Step.

Tap dance class was my favorite. Next to jazz. Next to ballet.

As a Renaissance woman, I did it all. Even outside of dance class, at home, I loved busting a move!

Turn up the Jock Jams, give me some pom poms and I choreographed quite the routine. And, of course, the long hallway between my bedroom and our family game room was the perfect place to leap, turn, spin, dosie doe and practice my dance recital routines.

Until the 3rd grade hit.

Cue: Me leaping and bounding like a Leprechaun down the runway upstairs.

Thump. Thump. Thump. Thump!

"Lauryn, what is that?! Are you ok? You sound like an elephant up there!"

I stopped dancing with happy feet.

A few weeks later, dance classes started back for the new school year at my "home away from home"— Shuffles Dance Studio, where I met my new ballet teacher Ms. Karen , a skinny blonde ex-professional ballerina—with thinning hair, protruding collar bones, and size negative A-sports dance leotards.

That first class back after the summer kicked my butt! Blame it on a summer spent eatings blue raspberry sno-cones by the poolside, enjoying Gold Fish crackers and apple juice at vacation bible school, and participating in story-writing camp—instead of doing dance camp—I definitely was not in dancing shape.

On the first class back in action, 10 of us "sugar plum fairies" quietly and admiringly looked to our fearless leader, Ms. Karen, as she walked us through a warm up sequence, beginning with "core work"—a completely new term to me.

Crunch. Crunch. Crunch. 100 reps later, I felt burning in my gut I'd never experienced before.

Our six-pack-abs sequence was then followed by some bar work, as Ms. Karen walked down the line, to gently correct our positions and form.

"Point and touch...and point and flex...point...and bend and snap..."

When she got to me, she pointed to my little back leotard tummy, full from my after-school snack of peanut butter crackers mom gave me in carpool on the way to dance: "Suck it in."

That night after class I told mom I didn't want to do ballet that year.

## FOURTH GRADE RECESS

*April 1997*

Fast forward about one month later to Fourth Grade recess.

I was 10 years old, with frizzy hair in a pink bow that Mom makes me wear. All I wanted to do was fit in.

The popular girls invited me to join their circle, gossiping about Melanie Strawn's ugly sweater and Eric Anderson's cute freckly face. Then the topic of weight came up.

The Queen Bee said, "Oh my gosh, you guys, I weighed myself last night, and I am sixty-nine pounds! I am soooo fat!" She looked at each of us in turn.

"What do you weigh?" One by one, we had to report to our drill sergeant.

At a healthy eighty pounds, I was by no means a fat kid, but when the circle got to me, I gulped and lied, "I don't know."

After school, I went home and stood in the pantry. Turning over my favorite Doritos snack pack, I began learning a whole new language—fat grams and calories. At age 10, my life path took a sharp turn.

# LOW-FAT YOGURT, ONE APPLE, THREE BABY CARROTS, A STICK OF GUM

*150 calories. Plus 80. Plus 12. Plus, 5 calories in that stick of gum.*

I meticulously scribbled inside my math notebook, pretending to pay attention to Mrs. Adams and her long-division problems on the whiteboard. After Dorito D-Day (the day my Dorito eating died), I became obsessed with counting calories and working them off twice as fast.

In a matter of months, I could have won any Quiz Bowl competition in macros. I knew the number of calories and fat grams in every single food on the shelf, as well as foods without labels—chicken, mashed potatoes, apples, carrots... you name it.

I was a trendsetter in this new diet: The fasting diet. My mom's brown sack lunches and napkin notes with hearts and smiley faces always ended up in the trash, and I quickly discovered that my chronic bloating also "magically" got better when I didn't eat.

That is, until the day I blacked out. Then I switched to vegetarian, vegan, South Beach, Atkins—whatever was popular at the time. PB & J's quickly got replaced by turkey, mustard, and lettuce—no cheese, please—on whole wheat diet bread. Then, just turkey.

*Protein revs your metabolism:* the cover of *Cosmopolitan* at the grocery store said so.

I often "accidentally" dropped my dinner roll or spaghetti meatballs on the floor for my dog, Bentley. When Mom asked if I wanted my favorite Rocky Road ice cream for dessert, I told her I was full (from not eating anything at all), and at Stephanie's 11th birthday sleepover, while everyone else ate pizza and cake, I excused myself to secretly eat the Zone Perfect Bar I'd stored in my duffel.

I also exercised whenever I could. *One more rep. One more rep. One more rep.* My internal Queen Bee drill sergeant constantly chased me. Squats in the shower. Jumping jacks during *Saved by the Bell* commercials. Running up and down the stairs in my house 20 times. A thousand crunches before breakfast. During basketball practice, I earned bonus points for running voluntary extra laps, and in dance, I snuck in a few extra calf raises for good measure.

The scale encouraged me to keep things going. Slowly but surely, I was making progress. Every morning at 6:15 a.m. and every night at 8:30 p.m., I reported to see if I had made weight for the day. Some days were better than others: down 0.8 ounces one day (*not bad*), another 0.2 ounces the next (*you better watch it*), the exact same the next (*no water!*), and then plummeting a drastic 1.2 pounds the next (*take that, no-budging scale!*)

These habits continued for several months, my new norm. That is, until the day I passed out in the shower.

## FEELING FAINT

The shower water was running. The room grew hazy. Very hazy.

"Lauryn, are you almost done? We need to get going. Lauryn? Lauryn!" The door crashed in, and Mom, hastily turning the water off, rushed to my side. "Lauryn, sweetheart. Wake up!" She pulled me out of the shower and onto the bathroom floor and wrapped me in a towel.

"Mom? What happened?" I asked groggily, slowly coming to.

"Sweetheart, I think you passed out in the shower. Are you okay? Sweetheart, what's wrong?" She hugged me tightly. "Have you eaten today? I don't think you've eaten anything today! Ashley? Ashley!"

"Please watch Lauryn," my mom told my sister as she rushed into the room at the sound of Mom's urgent calling. "I need to get her something to eat."

Just sixty seconds later, she was back. "Here, I brought you some peanut butter crackers. There are also some mini-muffins and juice! Eat this, and this." She cradled my head in her elbow and brought some peanut butter crackers shakily to my lips.

*May Day! May Day! Two hundred and ten calories! Two hundred and ten calories! Ten grams of fat! Ten grams of fat! This is going to blow my 0.5-gram limit for the day!*

These thoughts raced through my head, but I didn't feel good. I told my brain not to care about the calories for once. *I can burn it off later. I'll make up for it later.*

I slowly ate a cracker. Then a mini-muffin. Then I sipped from a Hi-C juice box.

"It's all going to be okay, it's all going to be okay," Mom said, her voice trembling with uncertainty.

## STICKERS & LOLLY POPS

A few hours after the shower incident, I found myself at my pediatrician's (Dr. Joe's) office in a cold, fluorescent lit shoe-box sized room that smelled like a combo pouparri, dirty diapers and peanut butter and jelly sandwiches.

The nurse poked and prodded me for stat bloodwork and urine sampling, took my blood pressure and temperature, asking my mom, "Has she always been this pale and tired looking?"—referring to those dark raccoon eye circles that had been with me for months.

"No, it's really just been the past several months it's seemed like something is off," mom replied. Her furrowed brows and tapping feet didn't help me feel at ease about the current situation.

Fifteen minutes later, Dr. Joe walked in and sat on his three-wheeled office stool.

"Well, no signs of strep or mono, but it does look like she is anemic and needs some fluids. How is she eating?" He asked.

If my refusal of a lolly pop at the end of the visit was any indication of the answer to that question, the truth was starting to come out.

Dr. Joe referred me to a specialist for an additional "workup" just to make certain everything else was ok.

## ANOREXIA

"You have anorexia," Dr. Portillo said.

*Ano-what? That sounds like an insect.*

"This is really serious. You could die from this."

*Die? From being thin and pretty and popular? Whatever.*

She powered on: "Your hair is falling out. You have anemia and mono. You've lost ten pounds in three months. Your body is shutting down."

*What is she talking about? This doctor's just trying to hijack my goals. There are tons of women who eat like I do and weigh less than me. They are pretty and fine.*

"Anorexia is really difficult to fight on your own. I'm recommending our intensive outpatient program—weekly appointments with a therapist, dietician, psychiatrist, myself, and group therapy. And, for now, you need to stop all exercise and outside activities to give your body a rest. If you continue to lose weight, then you'll have to go into the hospital. We need to get you healthy and keep you alive." She continued relentlessly, as if trying to cut through my internal admonitions.

*Can't hear you. Not listening. Not listening.*

She explained the game plan: Gain one pound per week, according to Dietician Tracy's "healthy eating" USDA Food Guidelines. This plan would entail eating twelve grains, three proteins, three vegetables, two fruits, three dairy exchanges, and three fats per day. No backsliding.

*I'm fine. This crazy doctor is freaking out for no reason. I'm going to be just fine. Everything is fine.*

## THE TREATMENT "SOLUTION"

I spent a total of four years of my life "behind bars"—living inside hospitals and treatment centers. My parents and siblings gave everything they had to keep me alive. Tears. Prayers. Encouragement. Fight. They remortgaged our "Leave it to Beaver" home three times to cover 1 million dollars of uninsured healthcare expenses so that I could see over fifty different specialists, all with similar prescriptions: Pop-Tarts, *more* pizza, *more* Prozac. Although they meant no harm, their common approach to healthy eating and restoration—symptom chasing—was far from the World Health Organization's definition of health: "A state of *complete* physical, mental and social well-being."

Just like the classic "symptom treating" advice for people who are overweight and obese—"you should just move more and eat less" (despite the fact that this strategy actually slows the metabolism more) or the classic "symptom treating" advice for people who have heartburn or constipation—"just take PPIs for the rest of your life" or "eat Fiber One bars" (not treating the root cause), my anorexia *symptoms* were often treated with what made the most sense for weight gain and food freedom: processed foods and selective serotonin reuptake inhibitor (SSRI) drugs, obviously.

The stakes to meet expectations and follow the rules were high.

# THE TWINKIE CHALLENGE

Then, there was the Twinkie challenge.

"Eat it." This was the first day of inpatient eating disorder treatment in Arizona. Now, at 12 years old, I'm on my own, 1,134 miles away from Mom and Dad, accelerating "adulting" to the collegiate level.

It was afternoon snack time: Twinkie versus Ding Dong. Which would you choose? You *must* choose one—no other option, at least for today. Over the next sixty days, I would get the opportunity to choose between Butterfinger and Snickers, banana split or caramel-fudge sundae, and tater tots or french fries.

Under the watchful gaze of the nurse, I reached for the Twinkie, an old childhood favorite. It felt like seemingly the lesser of two evils, with more sponge, less dark, and 150 calories versus the 160 calories in a Ding Dong. A better choice. Again, my inner monologue began to rationalize.

*You can work it off when you're out of here. You're going to work your butt off when you're outta here!*

The nurse put fifteen minutes on the clock, and the game began—telling my eleven new friends and me that if we wanted to get better, we'd leave no crumbs or cream behind. There was no way out. I couldn't hide it, toss it, or work off 150 calories on the StairMaster right after. I just had to sit there and eat it—every single crumb—as brain fog, headache, bloating, and stomach pain slowly set in.

There was no time to think or cry. A recovery coach pushed me to my first group therapy of the day: DBT, or dialectical behavior therapy, is a type of cognitive behavioral therapy with the goals of teaching people how to live in the moment, cope healthily with stress, regulate emotions, and improve relationships with others.

"How are we all feeling?" Barb, the therapist, opened the circle.

"Fat!" Cameron blurted.

"Triggered!" Annie piped in.

*Sick!* I thought. *How is this helping me get healthy?* Outwardly, I kept quiet. Barb simply smiled, letting the group get their thoughts off their chest.

A few hours after the Twinkie Challenge, shrimp fettuccine alfredo and garlic bread graced my plate, followed by a reappearance of Resource weight-gain ice cream for dessert—apparently a treatment staple. Amber hid her garlic bread in her sweatshirt: *a brilliant idea!* Tiffany refused dinner altogether. She got Ensured—two whole cans.

After dinner, the recovery coach locked the bathroom doors, and Nurse Susan dispensed TUMS and Lactaid pills to us girls, curled up in balls on the family room sofas. Our stomachs were writhing, digestive juices churning, and we felt as though bricks were sitting in our abdomens. The nurses turned on a Disney Channel show in an attempt to distract us; then, we retired upstairs for our five-minute monitored showers and evening bedtime routine.

Kimberly, a 17-year-old depressed anorexic, attempted to cut herself as the head recovery coach pinned her on the floor to get the razor out of her hands. Natalie, my 15-year-old roommate, shushed me as she threw up in her pillowcase while the scene with Kimberly was going down. Thirteen-year-old Carolyn snuck in a three-minute Jane-Fonda-inspired routine of jumping jacks, leg lifts, and crunches. By 10 p.m., the lights went out, and I slid under the covers, praying, *Lord, help me.*

I definitely wasn't in Kansas anymore.

Lots of symptom-chasing and treatment ensued.

## BIG BREASTS AND PROZAC

During another inpatient treatment stay, I remember an overweight Russian nutritionist told me she wanted to "plump me up and give me big breasts like hers." The psychiatrist on staff prescribed me anti-anxiety meds that took away my smile and a little spark, and my therapy sessions were primarily spent with me crying to go home.

Three months into it, I had put on about 25 pounds. I felt bloated, flat, inflamed yet again, and *still* obsessed with over-exercise and under-eating. In my mind, I wanted anything but what that treatment was teaching me.

## TUBED

At age 15, my pediatrician prescribed nightly tube feedings to "put weight on me." My sweet mom, desperate to keep me alive, would stick a nasal tube down my nose every night for my evening "meal"—a Nestle-sweetened chocolate formula delight.

Instead of hanging with friends in the Sonic drive-in parking lot after Friday night football games or going to the homecoming dance, my feeding tube and I had a hot date that started sharply at 9 p.m.

## PIZZA, PIZZA

*Stomach churning. Bubbling. Tooooooot. Embarrassed. Gassy.*

Pizza night—like every weekend for six months straight. Three slices of cheesy pepperoni pizza smiling back at me. Plus, a milkshake. Don't forget the slice of cheesecake.

I'm lactose and casein intolerant, but they didn't care. It was just my "disordered" brain speaking.

"Take this," the recovery coach said, handing me two Lactaid pills.

## EGG MCMUFFIN

Oh yes, and I will never forget Egg McMuffin Fridays in another center, although the staff told me it was just a breakfast sandwich. I believed this for weeks until the morning I woke up early to go to the bathroom and saw the recovery coach unwrapping McDonald's biscuits.

"Healthy eating" put me well on the way to chronic disease.

## ORTHOREXIA

Tired of fighting, my anorexia morphed. It transformed into orthorexia—the obsession with healthy eating—and I started eating again, only this time in a clean-eating form. I defined success through the accomplishment of a tough leg workout and cutting carbs. I ate according to a strict schedule and adhered to a bodybuilding diet, meticulously counting my carbs, fats, and proteins. My food and exercise rule list grew:

- No cooking with oils—use PAM;
- Eat every three hours;
- No sweet potatoes after noon and no eating after 8 p.m.;
- Drink a protein shake 30 minutes after a workout;
- Earn your carbs;
- No fruit;
- Never eat food from a restaurant;
- Pack your own food if you travel;

- Exercise six to eight hours per day—no excuses;
- Do cardio fasting—no eating for twelve hours before.

I was still stuck, still striving to be healthy and to just *feel good enough* in my own skin, until the day, at age 23, everything in me flashed back to that Fourth Grade recess that triggered my drive to lose weight.

## THE DAY MY WHOLE WORLD STOOD STILL

Four in the morning came too early: *Move it, move it, move it! You're wasting daylight. Time to get up. Drop and give me 100!*

Rolling out of bed, I did what I always did—every single morning: 100 flutter kicks, 100 leg raises, and 100 scissor kicks—they were my golden ticket to starting the day.

Eight minutes later, I bounded up off the floor and stumbled in the dark to my bathroom. Spit spot, I brushed my teeth, ran a straightener through my hair, slapped some blush on my pale face, and stepped on the scale. Like clockwork, I did this every morning, not thinking twice about it, just to check where I sat for the day. This morning, unlike any other morning over the past thirteen years, brought a new reality to the surface: the scale read 79 pounds.

*Really? That can't be right.*

This was a number I had not seen since I was 10 years old, when all of this daily drill-sergeant craziness had begun. This, I felt, was a number reserved for starving women and men in Africa, anorexics in a hospital bed, or Twiggy models.

*I am over this anorexia thing,* I thought.

Reflecting on the past several weeks, I knew I hadn't been feeling well. I had difficulty breathing and very sharp chest pains. I had to clench my chest to get through them when they came. I suffered through horrific, knife-stabbing stomach aches, leaving me doubled over in pain. This was joined by unrelenting diarrhea after every meal I ate and perpetuating fatigue and weakness. I had been seeing spots or blacking out after a mile sprint on the treadmill or sometimes even just walking up the stairs to my apartment.

Something hadn't been right.

*But what did this all mean?*

Brushing my fear and shock to the side, I resolved in my eternally optimistic mind that today could be—would be—when I changed things for myself. Five minutes later, I was out the door. I had a protein shaker with eight ounces of water, a scant scoop of protein powder meticulously measured, and a new, health-oriented game plan: Hit it hard in the gym. Then refuel with a hearty breakfast of twelve almonds (two more than my usual ten) sprinkled with cinnamon and a double scoop of more protein powder in water to help me start to get healthier again.

For each day, I marked 4:45 a.m. to 7:45 a.m. on my calendar as my first workout of that day. Three hours to make my dream body happen before sitting four hours in my morning grad school classes, pining for my next hour-long workout fix in the gym on campus during my lunch break.

Peeling out of my driveway, I took a left, heading toward my YMCA gym, when I hit the first stoplight. I remembered that I had planned on starting my routine off with the StairMaster that morning. Quickly making a turn, I headed right, determined to get a great sweat in on the third machine from the left in the row of four. It was the newest machine, and level twenty gave off the fastest-paced workout of them all. I also hoped my StairMaster routine would dispel the stress I felt about that darned scale—maybe it was broken? Seventy-nine pounds, really?—and began to pep myself up with my eternally positive mindset: *you can do this.*

As I drove, I prayed. Out loud.

"God, help me kick this today. Help me kick this in the butt! Give me the strength, the power, to make a change. I want to be well. I want to be strong. I want to be healthy! I want the courage to add a tablespoon of almond butter or a couple more almonds to my breakfast. And help me to step for thirty minutes less on my StairMaster than usual."

Little did I know what was in store. Zooming into the YMCA parking lot, I parked my car near the doors by the StairMasters. Hopping out, I popped my trunk to grab the stack of eight different *Oxygen* and *Fitness* magazines stowed in two large Lululemon bags (the same issues I grabbed every morning and read, then read again, for the latest diet tips and workouts during my first 45-minute cardio warm-up, and my second 45-minute cardio cooldown after hitting the weights).

Before I could even shut the trunk and head inside, I felt a hand touch the back of my shoulder.

"Good morning, Lauryn. How are you today?"

I span around sharply in surprise and saw seven fellow gym-goers surrounding me: Suzy, Louise, Andy, Bob, Johnny, Tanya, and Judith—individuals I had seen every morning at 5 a.m. at the YMCA over the past year, ranging in age from 30 to the mid-50s.

"Good morning?" I said, confusion clear in my voice.

"Lauryn, you've been in our hearts. We can't let you go in there today," Louise said abruptly, taking a step closer to me. "We're worried about you," she added. "We all came together this morning because we all felt like we just had to say something."

Andy spoke up, "We've seen you every day for the past year, but especially over the past several months, we've been worried about you. It seems like you're getting thinner and thinner, weaker. You don't seem healthy. We don't want anything to happen to you."

"What? I'm fine," I said defensively.

"We're worried you might collapse, Lauryn," Suzy chimed in, voice quaking. "That you're going to be on that StairMaster and have a heart attack. We don't want to see that happen."

"For some reason," Louise said, "God really put you in our hearts, all of our hearts. We hadn't even spoken to each other until yesterday. We came here together outside the Y this morning to give you this message—we want to help you out."

I was shocked, speechless.

"We want to take you to Vanderbilt's ER," Bob said. "Have them check you out. Just do a physical. Make sure everything is okay. If they say you're fine, it will put us at ease."

My head pinged like a pinball as I looked from one talking head to another. I gripped my keys tightly and clung to my magazines. I could feel fire flaming in my eyes. A lump welled in my throat.

"No, thank you all, but no, thank you. I'm seeing a doctor and taking care of myself." This was a lie; I rarely saw my doctor. "You're all so kind to worry, but really, I'm fine."

I took a step toward the YMCA door, and the group of seven huddled closer around me.

"Lauryn, we're sorry, but we're not giving you an option today. You need to go with us," Louise said. I looked again at each of these seven individuals, basically seven strangers. There was fear and pain in their faces. The situation no longer involved just my parents speaking up from 350 miles away—still thinking, praying, fighting, and eating for me daily. I thought back to the prayer I had spoken aloud in the car just minutes before pulling into the YMCA and suddenly knew I didn't have a choice.

I took a deep breath. I unclenched my keys and loosened my grip on my magazines. Tears welled in my eyes.

I surrendered.

*It will be okay. I'll just get checked out, and I'll do my workout later this afternoon, then again tonight. It will be okay. Just a check-up. Not the hospital.*

I hated the hospital.

*Thank you, Lord,* I prayed. *Thank you for reaching out. Maybe, just maybe, this is what I just prayed for—the start of something new.*

## 48 HOURS LATER: CODE BLUE!

Beep. Beep. Beeeeeep! Beeeeeep!

"Lauryn...? Lauryn...? Lauryn!" My mom's voice rang out as she nudged me, the sense of panic clear in her shrill tone.

*What is happening...?*

My heart rate plummeted: 35... 33... 32... 31...

"Code Blue! Code Blue! Code Blue!" The nurse yelled over the intercom, and three nurses rushed into the hospital room.

"Lauryn!" My mom called out as she was moved to one side.

*What's all the commotion about?* I thought to myself, confused and unaware.

"We've got a coder on our hands!" One nurse phoned a doctor on her walkie-talkie.

"Sweetheart, Lauryn... wake up, wake up!" My mom's voice called over the commotion.

"What's happening?!" Dad said. "Oh my God, oh my God, oh my God... No, Lord, please no."

The doctor rushed in to assess the situation.

"Let's move her."

Another nurse signaled the CCU—the critical care unit—to come to take me off the general ward.

"She's not stable."

Everyone was blurry and moved in slow motion, but something inside me felt an odd sense of peace. A calm, assured, hopeful voice whispered in my heart:

*You're going to be okay. Just buckle up because it's going to be a bumpy ride. It's time to wring this eating disorder and take your life back.*

*Lightbulb: health is an inside job.*

# MCDONALD'S MACROS

As you might have guessed, treatment ensued. The next four weeks were "fun-filled"—feeding tubes, heart rate monitors, and IV fluids followed by another twelve months spent in yet *another* treatment center in Miami.

My ten-count almond and protein shake breakfast turned into Honey Nut Cheerios Tuesdays, double bagel Wednesdays, and Egg McMuffin Fridays. My frozen turkey patty and steamed broccoli dinners morphed into pizza and milkshakes. Grad school pursuits were replaced with daily therapy sessions and group work spent talking, and talking, and talking about the eating disorder nonstop.

Same story. But, unlike all the other times in my treatment to date, something inside me had changed. Often, we don't know how good we can feel until we feel good or *really* bad.

I made up my mind that, no matter how bloated, anxious, self-conscious, or stuck I felt going through the treatment motions, *there's got to be another way*. There is another way.

No matter how crappy I felt eating rubbery eggs and fake cheese on crusty biscuits or how much my lactose intolerance acted up after slurping chocolate milkshakes alongside three large slices of pepperoni pizza, life was going to be different on the other side. No more extremes. No more rules. No more "good" or "bad" foods.

I also knew that if I wanted healing—true healing—it would not come from green juice, calorie counters, an elimination diet, the USDA Guidelines, or a Twinkie Challenge. To date, no one diet, fad, rule, or symptom-chasing approach to "fixing" my body has been the answer to healing and feeling well.

Although I was not a hundred percent sure of what that answer was yet, during this time, the Lord reminded me of a verse I had read while in my hospital bed thirteen years earlier— my first time in a hospital bed: *"For I know the plans I have for you. Plans to prosper you. Not harm you. Plans to give you hope and a future."*

*I will recover*, I vowed.

## POST-RECOVERY RECOVERY

Life on the other side of diet slavery is pretty great. I got my mind back. I got my life back. That said, life was not all rainbows and butterflies in the post-recovery years, far from it.

Chronic dieting and disordered eating wreak havoc on your health, both during the time you struggle and the years after. "Post-recovery recovery" is the term I have coined for the side effects that can happen to the body after years of not treating it well—be it disordered eating, processed food eating, restrictive eating, binging and purging, chronic cardio, and beyond.

Many healthcare professionals, treatment programs, diet protocols, or books about diet rarely address the chronic health side effects that arise from long-term restrictive diets, particularly if individuals look fine on the outside or are free of official mental health diagnoses.

This was me.

By age 29, I joined the nearly 90 percent of Americans with at least one chronic disease (1). Only, in my case, that number surpassed ten.

Doctors diagnosed me with (brace yourself, it's quite the list): Colitis, Osteoporosis, Anxiety, Celiac Disease, Hashimoto's, Lupus, Reactivated Epstein-Barr Virus, Diabetes, Chronic Migraines, Lyme Disease, Mycotoxin Illness, and Mast Cell Activation Syndrome.

Both my "healthy eating" during my dieting days *and* eating disorder treatment destroyed my health.

With this lengthy list of diagnoses came dozens of referrals to specialists. There were gastroenterologists, endocrinologists, neurologists, rheumatologists, cardiologists, and more. I found myself in the ER more than a handful of times with a variety of wild symptoms—from air hunger to heart-attack-like chest pains, dizziness, nausea, numbness and tingling, and hypoglycemic episodes—that heart rate monitors, basic CBC blood panels, and even CAT scans could not pinpoint. Medical expenses from doctors, emergency room visits, urgent care trips, MRI and CT scans, and supplements easily exceeded a hundred thousand dollars.

How could I—a healthy, young, fit nutritionist and functional medicine practitioner, doing all the "right things"—drinking water, taking probiotics, eating green things, and talking about healthy living, go from seemingly fine one day to chronically ill? My healthy habits should have made me feel better, not worse.

No doctor—conventional and holistic alike—could explain it either. They scratched their heads. Many told me they had never seen a case like mine, as they continued to pass me on to the next specialist in town to try to solve the puzzle. Some white lab coats prescribed steroids; others prescribed hormones. Others—including Dr. Internet—of course, told me to take boatloads of supplements and eat a Low FODMAP, low carb, low histamine, autoimmune paleo diet...

However, did you know that **long-term restrictive diets and "green allopathy"** are just as bad for your gut health as processed foods (2)?

In my case, I lost 20 unwanted pounds in a matter of months and was limited to only five to ten foods because that was all my body could handle.

Sweet potatoes gave me brain fog. Spinach gave me IBS. Nuts and ground beef made me constipated. Broccoli exacerbated by colitis. Dark chocolate triggered shortness of breath.

I felt stuck, perhaps like many of you have felt when "healthy eating" protocols or healthcare are not working, or when it seems like no matter how hard you try, I felt like my body was working against me.

What I soon learned, and what many of my doctors did not understand, was that something deeper was going on "underneath the hood"—something inside my *second brain.*

*Something had to change.*

## HEALTH IS AN INSIDE JOB

Fast forward one last time—now age 33. Same exact predicament I'd been 10 years earlier: flat on my back, in a hospital bed, in the ER, feeling like I was having a heart attack.

By this time, the Mayo Clinic had turned me away. The Cleveland Clinic passed me from specialist to specialist with NO conclusion.

And what was even more frustrating: I was doing all the things to be healthy— eating right, working out, avoiding gluten and sugar. But it still wasn't working.

And all I hoped and prayed for is that someone would take the time to really figure out the root causes that were going on under the hood.

Dr. Hung, an overnight physician resident, frazzled from juggling 10 other patients in the packed ER, walked in, looked at my chart and delivered the bad news:

"Lauryn, I know you feel like this is serious...But according to your labs, as far as we can tell, everything is normal..."

Then he added: "You know Lauryn, there are times conventional medicine will fail you, this is one of them."

And, in that moment, something inside me flickered, "NO MORE!" And a lightbulb went off: HEALTH IS AN INSIDE JOB!

All these years, they'd been missing the link, and I was going to figure it out.

## FEELING GOOD IS YOUR BIRTHRIGHT

Nothing changes in our lives or health *until* we **change our second brain**. Not our diet. Not more supplements.

This isn't woo-woo talk. This is science, which is why we are here today and why you are reading this book.

Although there is no one-size-fits-all approach to anyone's health optimization journey, if there's one thing you'll hear me repeat time and time, it is this:

> ***When given the right tools, your body wants to innately heal itself.***

So let's give it those right tools!

# PART ONE: GUT HEALTH FUNDAMENTALS

# CHAPTER 1:
# A POP-TART EPIPHANY

Do you remember your first "most embarrassing moment?" You know, that time in your life when you first realized what sticking out feels like?

For me, it happened when I was six. I was spending the summer at Vacation Bible School. I remember it vividly: it had been a long day building up a sweat and playing with my friends. When we finally sat down for circle story time, I... well... I let one rip right in front of my crush.

"Lauryn tooted!" another 6-year-old whispered in that 6-year-old whisper everyone could hear.

As I immediately grew red-faced, the other kids in the classroom burst out in laughter as they diverted away from me to the outer edges of the carpet—leaving me alone in the middle, like Pumba in *The Lion King*. And the look my crush gave me told me it was safe to say that he found me gross.

I wanted to crawl into a hole. I was embarrassed, completely ashamed of my body. How could I trust it? From that moment on, my body (and my gut) were not on the best of terms.

Which is precisely why we are here today. We are here to talk about a big problem that has festered within our current health and diet culture. We are here to talk about a solution to that problem.

Have you ever wanted to change something about your body but struggled to do so? It seems as if no matter what you try and how hard you try, your body is working against you.

Have you wanted to lose or gain those last 5–10 pounds? Clear up your skin? Have you wanted to say goodbye to migraines, hair loss, or fatigue that no amount of coffee will touch?

Maybe you've tried cutting out carbs, meat, and fat or eating bacon and butter together in a saturated fat binge. You've Google searched for the best skin creams, rubbed ROGAINE® on your scalp, or maybe even eaten a Pop-Tart for a boost of sugar (because obviously, chasing symptoms makes sense), which is exactly like what happened that day during my own Pop-Tart epiphany.

## THE POP-TART EPIPHANY

My Pop-Tart epiphany came on the second day—my first morning—of inpatient eating disorder treatment at the Children's Hospital.

At 7:30 a.m., the nurse entered and placed a meal tray on my bedside table.

"Breakfast is served. Let's see what you have here!" She chimed with that irritating morning cheeriness that nobody wants to hear first thing in the morning, least of all a grumpy 10-year-old. The purple checklist she lifted from the tray noted the foods included in my breakfast. Peeking beneath the lid covering a plate, she called out each item.

"Chocolate milk, banana, cottage cheese, toaster pastries. Looks like it's all here. Eat up!" Staring at the heavily processed toaster pastries, I felt a lump form in my throat. Tears stung my eyes, and fear rose in my belly.

"Do I need to eat all this? Two whole packs of toaster pastries? That's four whole pastries!" Even to a 10-year-old, that seemed wrong.

"Yup. That's what it says right here on this list—two toaster pastries. Eat them." The smile was still glued to her face. It bordered on scary, amplified by the fear I felt at my alien surroundings at the ominous plate of food before me.

My stomach was in knots. I wanted to break out of there, but there was no escape, no way out. This was, and in many cases still is, how it goes in the hospital when you have an eating disorder.

Nurse Betty, who reminds me now of Professor Umbridge from *Harry Potter*, plopped down in the recliner chair, whipped out the latest issue of *People* magazine, and put her feet up.

"You have thirty minutes to eat," she said sternly. "Last night, the staff left a note saying you tried to get by leaving with some gravy on your tray. This time, make sure there's not a crumb left."

Never in my life had I eaten four toaster pastries in one sitting. Even when I did eat such food, it was a single frosted strawberry pastry. Looking at Nurse

Betty, I gulped as I dropped a slow, solitary nod. A tear slid down my cheek. Hands trembling, I tore open the silver wrapping on the first pack and peeled the clear plastic from a bruised half-banana and a bowl of clumpy cottage cheese.

Biting into the banana mush, taking a forkful of chunky, slimy cottage cheese, I thought that if I focused on getting these foods down, maybe that stack of pastries would disappear. The clock ticked off the seconds as I washed the banana and cheese down with chocolate milk.

"Fifteen minutes," the nurse warned, looking up from her magazine. I wondered what would happen if I failed to eat the stack in front of me. My mind conjured up images of force-feeding and other horrors.

I hadn't touched the pastries. I considered that maybe one of the syrupy sweet nutrition shakes was worth it. I had heard stories on my first day about the so-called punishment drinks the nurses dished out when a patient refused food.

In my head, I gave myself a pep talk: *It's not worth it. They'll think you're a horrible patient. They will keep you here longer. They will threaten to "tube" you.* I kept telling myself I could do it, that when I got out of the hospital, I could go right back to skipping meals, running laps, and doing a million jumping jacks. But now, I needed to eat. Picking up the first of the four pastries, I bit into the hard crust again and again, slowly at first, and then I focused on getting through all four.

Ten minutes later, with a gurgling stomach and the beginnings of bloat and impending constipation, the deed was done.

"Get it," the nurse said, pointing out a crumb hiding in the corner of the tray. I duly obliged. "Good, you made it in time. Now you can read or use points to watch some TV." TV was available on a strict point-based system. Later, I could go to the Teen Room for crafts and see Mom and Dad, but only if I ate everything on my tray—nutrition shakes did not qualify. But at that moment, I could feel that something was very wrong, and I needed to go to the bathroom.

"I don't feel good," I said.

"You were told the rules. No bathroom for at least thirty minutes after eating," Nurse Betty barked. That was the rule to prevent girls from purging.

"But I really don't feel good," I said, now with a hint of desperation in my voice.

"Just lie in bed. I'll get something for your tummy." She turned and walked away.

Still in bed, my legs hugged tightly to my chest; I could feel my stomach gurgling as shooting, stabbing, piercing pains shot through my abdomen. My gut sounded like a cauldron bubbling over a fire.

"Please, God, help me," I whispered, breathing through the storm inside. I felt like a prisoner inside my own body, like there was no way out.

And then, I felt the warm, watery stool oozing out all over the bed. I was exasperated, defeated. My stomach still churned, but at least there was some relief. Crying, I pressed the nurse-call button for help.

"Can I help you?" a fuzzy radio voice came through the speaker.

"I just went to the bathroom, all over myself." My face felt red hot with shame. I knew they would give me the nutrition shake or a feeding tube now because I'd lost all that food I'd just eaten. Suddenly Nurse Betty ran back into my room.

"Honey, what did you do? What happened?" I cried buckets. I didn't know what to say. As she took in the scene, her face turned from worry to disgust.

"This is disgusting," she said, scowling. "First, let's clean you up, then the bed, and then, we're getting a doctor in here. This is unacceptable! You're going to have to make up for this," she yelled, wagging her finger at me. She left to get towels and cleaning supplies.

Half an hour later, I was showered, dressed, and back in a fresh bed with a 350-calorie Ensure nutritional shake on my bedside tray and 30 minutes back on the clock. After I finished the shake, I sank back under the covers, praying it would all go away.

Beneath the hum of the fluorescent light behind my bed, I watched the clock tick off seconds, minutes, and hours. I thought about going back to school, about being away from the hospital, back in fifth grade with my friends, when rude nurses and crusty toaster pastries would fade into bad memories.

*Somewhere in my 10-year-old brain, a light bulb flickered: our inside affects our outside and how we feel. If our gut doesn't feel good, we don't feel good.*

## IMPROVING YOUR HEALTH STARTS FROM THE INSIDE OUT

This epiphany was the first time I connected the dots to a bigger story that would later become the story of my life for the next two decades–the story of how what we eat (and what we digest) impacts our total health; and how the extremes of any diet – be they found in Pop-Tarts or protein bars–are not the answer to getting well, and staying well.

While my example may sound extreme, it is not far from the countless stories of others who have experienced a symptomatic, medicated, supplemental, or diet-based approach to treating their odd signs and symptoms.

Feed the girl with "eating problems" Pop-Tarts, pizza, and Prozac.

Give Buddy the low-fat whole-grain Cheerios and a statin drug to lower his elevated cholesterol.

Jacob's got ADHD? Lifelong Ritalin and purportedly healthier snacks like fruit gummies and strawberry (still sugar-loaded) yogurt to the (supposed) rescue!

Becky can't lose weight, no matter how healthy she eats or how much she works out. More cardio, intermittent fasting, and no more than 20 net carbs per day should set her body straight.

As for Sarah's recurring candida and small intestinal bacterial overgrowth protocol: a low-carb diet, followed by a bone-broth-only fast, then an autoimmune paleo diet, and then a carnivore's diet; oh yes, and anti-microbial and anti-fungal herbs, nystatin, coffee enemas, juices. Something's eventually got to work!

All of these treatments, protocols, and prescriptions to optimize your body, with little to no results. What gives?

The answer: eating healthily may not be the solution—at least, not how you think.

Instead, the solution for radically transforming our health lies within our stress-response systems and our gut microbiomes. These are the gateways to health. They're the gateways to our immune system—helping us combat pathogens, viral infections, toxins, disease, and illness, or, if managed incorrectly, making us susceptible to them.

To help you understand how the gut microbiome affects your health, consider the following:

**Physically, your gut determines your metabolism and weight:** Mice given gut bacteria from obese subjects gain weight, whereas mice that get bacteria from lean subjects lose weight, with no change in their diet or exercise (3).

**The gut is responsible for 70 to 80 percent of your immune system**—acting like a bouncer for cancer growth, acne, and food intolerances.

**The gut drives your cravings and blood sugar:** People who hate broccoli are called Super Tasters because they have specific gut bugs that make it taste bitter (4). Chocolate lovers have gut bugs that crave sweets (5).

**The gut *is* your second brain:** Have you ever experienced butterflies in your stomach? Boom: Gut-brain connection! There are over 500 million neurons–brain cells–inside your gut alone, and 80 percent of all messages–the thoughts you think, the symptoms you feel, and how your body operates–are actually delivered between the gut and the brain.

*Translation: your gut is kind of a big deal, and health is an inside job.*

When you improve your second brain, *your whole health can change!*

If you've struggled with lingering symptoms, food bondage, or mystery health conditions, then this book is for you.

Likewise, this is also a book for my fellow clinicians and practitioners who work with patients and clients. This book is for healers who understand there is *more* behind the cause of chronic illness than a Ritalin, Prozac, or statin-drug deficiency and who understand that the underlying mechanisms (especially the gut-brain connection) play a critical role in helping their patients reset, not just manage, the chronic-disease epidemic.

This book is for those who are "doing all the things" to be healthy, like drinking green juice, popping supplements, eating low-fat diets, high-fat diets, plant-based diets, all-meat diets, elimination diets, and everything in between, but despite "doing all the things," you've discovered something is still not working. Something is missing to feel optimal. In some cases, you may even feel worse.

Lastly, this is a book for those health enthusiasts, Dr. Google searchers, and wellness warriors who have heard and know that the gut-brain connection is *important* and *want* to be healthy but, to be honest, are overwhelmed with all the noise out there. If this is you, you've come to the right place.

Hippocrates, the father of medicine, once said that "all disease begins in the gut." I say *all wellness* begins in the gut too.

# CHAPTER 2:
# WHY YOUR GUT MATTERS

Health is an inside job. Both mentally and physically. While you *may* still survive if your inside health is not optimal, only the strongest will thrive.

Your greatest weapon? Your gut—the second brain.

Gut health is the new black, a hot topic. Everyone is talking about it.

Unless you've been living under a rock, you're probably no stranger to the gut health buzz.

From probiotics and kombucha to bone broth and collagen probiotic-enriched skin creams, such products continue to grow in popularity, as does the realization that impeccable gut health is one of the best health insurance plans you can have over the course of your lifetime.

To highlight this surge in popularity, between 2010 and 2015, there were only 180,086 studies published on PubMed dedicated to the term "gut microbiome." However, between 2015 and 2021, there were over 1,762,000 studies released—more than a 900 percent increase. New headlines are released daily, supporting the connections between gut health and total body health. Good gut health is touted as the modern day's all-purpose cleaner—a panacea.

So, what do "bad gut health" and "good gut health" actually mean? And why is "good gut health" so crucial for our total health anyway? After all, it seems far-fetched to claim that good gut health results in clearer skin, mental clarity, good libido, a sleek physique, and less susceptibility to viruses like the common cold and flu.

When you realize how the gut works, you realize that systemic inflammation, immune activation, and even how you think, deal with anxiety, and see the world are all rooted in the gut.

## THE GUT-IMMUNE-BRAIN CONNECTION

Seventy to eighty percent of your immune cells (6) are produced and housed in the gut alone, which is why your mom's homemade chicken noodle soup–gut-healing bone broth–was always the cure for the common cold. If your gut gets inflamed, what do you think happens to your immune system? *Exactly.*

Your gut and your brain are also directly connected by way of the vagus nerve, making your gut the "second brain." In fact, I argue that it should really be called the "first brain" since it contains more than 100 million nerve cells and dictates every mental and physical process in your body, including birthing new neurons in your brain itself through the metabolism produced when it processes foods such as potatoes (glucose), salmon (proteins), and avocado (fatty acids).

The brain and gut talk to each other on a two-way street. Even if you don't perceive something to be stressful or brain-activating in the moment, the news you consume, the endless social media scrolls, the grapples you get into, and the conversations you hold send signals to the gut. These signals may be either inflammatory or anti-inflammatory, activating your immune system for better or worse. A virus of the mind can be a virus of the body and vice versa.

Your gut-lining tissues, digestive organs, *and* gut bacteria serve as the gatekeepers for all exposures we encounter on a daily basis, keeping pathogens, antigens, and toxins out of your bloodstream, cells, and tissues while allowing nutrients, vitamins, and minerals in—that is, as long as your gut is in tip-top shape.

Suppose there is a defect in the balance of your gut bacteria, your gut lining tissues, your digestive process, or the way you perceive the world. In that case, inflammation, disease, and an immune cascade arise.

To fully understand this concept, let's take a short trip back to Ninth Grade Biology and review a few gut health fundamentals (and fill in a few gaps that your science teacher didn't originally teach).

## NINTH-GRADE BIOLOGY

"Today, we're going to talk all about the human digestive system," Mrs. Castleberry says enthusiastically in Grade Nine Biology class. "*Digestion* is necessary to break a complex mixture of proteins, carbohydrates, lipids, and other substances into small molecules, which can move through cell membranes. It takes place in the alimentary canal, a continuous tube running from the mouth to the anus. And..."

Admit it; she lost you at "anus." At least, she did me. The remainder of her painful sixty-minute lecture sounds more like Snoopy from an episode of *Charlie Brown*, so naturally, you begin daydreaming about Aaron's dreamy smile, the names of your three children, and whatever other fancies you have pop up in your brain.

Sixty minutes later, the bell rings, and you break free. You manage to make it through "Unit 6: Digestion" on your own, cramming for the quiz that Friday to regurgitate terms like "hydrolysis," "mucus," "pharynx," and "bile" before moving on to "Unit 7: Hormones & Reproduction."

*Chapter closed—end of the story.*

Unfortunately, this is the extent of most people's experience with learning about the digestive system and gut health. Even in medical school and allied healthcare education, the central role that the gut microbiome plays in total human health is largely unaddressed. The average most up-to-date medical textbook is already outdated by three years, meaning by the time your doctor exits their four-year program, they may be at least twelve years behind the latest research.

Before 1910 (the year that the Flexner Report (7) was released—a report that mandated medical education completely abandon complementary and holistic medicine), medical education and practice looked to Hippocratic philosophy as a guiding light, emphasizing natural forces within us as the true healers of disease. Not medicine. Not insurance coverage. Not the food guide pyramid. Natural forces *within* us.

In Ancient Greece and Rome, disease was understood as *dis-ease*, or physical imbalance. Medical intervention, therefore, was purposed with the goal of the restoration of harmony rather than the waging of a war against disease. In the prevention and treatment of disease in classical medicine, food, diet, and digestive health was king.

I have had the honor to work with many amazing healthcare professionals, and many have come to me as patients and clients with various gut-related ailments themselves, including Irritable Bowel Disease (IBS), low energy, autoimmune disease, brain fog, migraines, acne, stubborn body fat, infertility, and insomnia. "Why didn't they teach us this in school?" most of them say.

These were my thoughts exactly when I first realized the impact of my own gut health on how I felt—both inside and outside of my gut.

## CRYSTAL LIGHT CONUNDRUM

"Hi, I'm Lauryn, and I am a Crystal Light Addict."

This is what I would have told you if you had met me when I was 22. I would have Crystal Light with breakfast, Crystal Light with lunch, and Crystal Light with dinner; artificially sweetened, Strawberry-Orange-Banana powdery goodness, please!

Never mind the bloating, gas, constipation, brain fog, "hangry" appetite, and headaches accompanying my daily cocktails. I never correlated them with my beverage consumption. Those woeful experiences were my norm—just as eating Big Macs, a reliance on coffee-dependent energy, and experiencing allergies and headaches are many people's day-to-day normal.

Drinking Crystal Light every day was *my* norm until the day I inadvertently ran out of Crystal Light. For the first time in a long time, I had no Crystal Light with my breakfast, no Crystal Light with my lunch, and no Crystal Light with my dinner that day. Surprisingly, I had no bloating, gas, constipation, brain fog, or headache. *Hm. That's strange.*

However, I didn't correlate them with my Crystal Light consumption. This could have been innocent overlooking, but I suspect that this initial inability to connect the dots came from a subconscious refusal to acknowledge my problem. To compensate for my loss, I stocked up on eight tubs of the magic potion at the grocery store the next day and drank two 40 oz Nalgene bottles full of the stuff.

By 5 p.m., I was curled over in the fetal position on the floor, feeling a knife-like stabbing in my gut. All those symptoms that accompanied every meal returned in a way that I had never experienced. That day, I learned the hard way that additives and chemicals were not my friends.

On this day, the lightbulb again lit up: *health is an inside job*. The experience inspired me to learn more and pursue my education further. Fast-forward a few years later to the day-one lecture of nutrition school on stomach acid, when my former Crystal Light conundrum finally made sense.

# NUTRITION SCHOOL DAY-ONE LESSON: BLOATING, GAS, CONSTIPATION, BRAIN FOG, AND HEADACHES ARE *NOT* NORMAL

"Who's experienced bloating or indigestion before?" Cathy, the Nutrition 101 instructor, asked the class.

All 46 students raised their hands.

"Did you know that bloating and heartburn are often triggered by low stomach acid and low digestive enzyme production?" Cathy said. "If you want to test this theory for yourself, today at lunch, take a little challenge: the HCl digestive enzymes stomach acid challenge. It's really simple. Here are the steps:

"*Step 1*: Before you eat, take one or two HCl digestive enzymes with your meal. This is a hydrochloric acid tablet, similar to the stomach acid you should *already* have in your stomach, but most people are deficient in it. Then wait a minute.

"*Step 2*: If you don't feel a slight warming sensation, take one more tablet, and wait. The goal is to try to experience a warming sensation.

"*Step 3*: Once you feel a slight warming sensation in your gut, you know you've found your therapeutic dose. Over time, as you continue to work on improving your gut health as a whole, you will find that your natural stomach acid kicks up, and you'll need less and less HCl to support digestion."

So, lunchtime came around, and I had a grilled chicken breast, broccoli, and sweet potato—a pretty innocent meal. Typically, any meal required me to pop two TUMS afterward; I experienced bloating after nearly every meal.

*Here goes nothing*, I thought, popped the tablets, waited for that warm feeling, and, when it came, I ate my lunch. And then, I waited. I waited for the bloating, for the pain, a pain which, like magic, never came. No bloating, no energy dip, no brain fog. I was elated, happy, and *comfortably full.*

*Aha,* I thought. Support your digestion, and how you *feel* totally changes.

# DIGESTION BASICS

Your gut is the gateway to your health. Did you know that:

- **Seventy to eighty percent of your immune cells (T cells or "Tregs") are located in your gut** (8) and can be manipulated with diet, nutrition, and lifestyle, acting like a bouncer for cancer growth, acne, and food intolerances (which is why people who eat green things, exercise and hit spin class, sleep well, and do not smoke are said to be "healthier").
- **Your gut is your largest endocrine hormone-producing organ**—producing over thirty hormones and regulating your monthly cycle, energy levels, and ability to build strength and gain muscle thyroid, estrogen, cortisol, and testosterone levels (9–12).
- **Ninety percent of your serotonin (your "feel good" mood-boosting chemicals) are produced in your gut**—responsible for your emotions and how you feel (13), explaining why clinical depression goes into remission when study subjects supplement with high-dose probiotics and why a good morning poo makes you feel amazing!
- **The gut drives your cravings and blood sugar.** I have already mentioned Super Tasters and how gut bugs heavily influence your cravings, giving you the scientific evidence you needed to justify why you reached for the brownie—*they made you do it!*
- **The gut is called your "second brain" because it contains 500 million neurons**—that's *more* brain cells in your microbiome than any other part of your peripheral nervous system. Additionally, your vagus nerve–the nerve that controls the mechanics of digestion–is *directly connected* from your frontal lobe to your gut. Also, the gut influences your brain. Eighty percent of all messages–the thoughts you think and symptoms you feel–are actually delivered *from* the gut *to* the brain.
- **Your gut microbiome influences your cravings and metabolism.** Overgrown strains or pathogenic gut bacteria may crave foods you are intolerant to or make you feel unwell. Most of your ghrelin (the hunger hormone that facilitates fat storage and regulates body weight) is produced in the gut mucosa. Furthermore, certain gut bacteria harvest more calories than others—explaining why some people are leaner and others heavier (14–17).

# YOUR HEALTH HIERARCHY OF NEEDS (STARTS IN YOUR GUT)

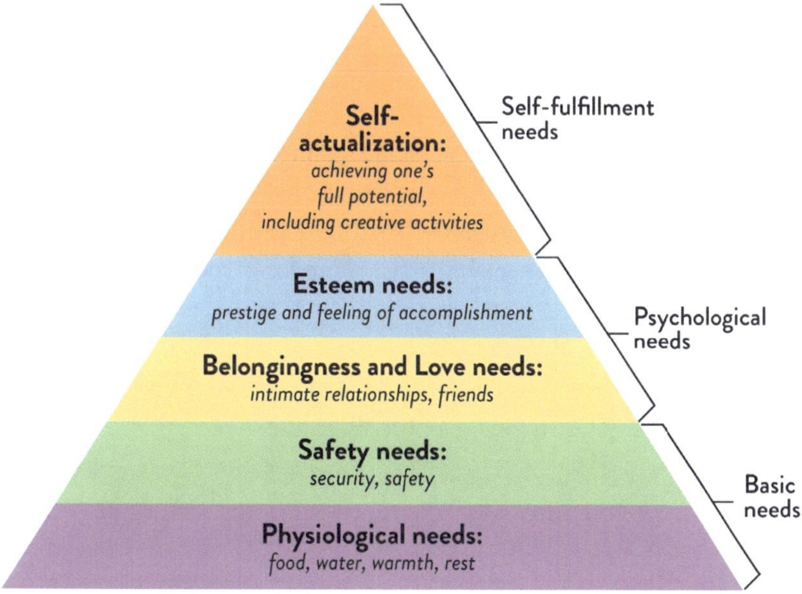


If you have ever taken a psychology class, you are probably familiar with Maslow's Hierarchy of Needs.

Maslow's Hierarchy of Needs is a theory that details the basic requirements all humans need to thrive. You may even have encountered it at work, with it widely being used as a motivational model to help managers and leaders understand how to motivate their people.

According to Maslow's theory, your basic human needs are arranged in a pyramid, with some needs–such as physiological needs–being more basic than others, such as relationship needs. In order to climb the hierarchy towards "self-actualization," or fulfilling your life purpose, your bottom needs *must* be met first. In essence, you must first ensure that you have the right conditions for your survival, including your health, safety, and security, to have the will and the motivation to work up the hierarchy and develop in the image of what you want to achieve.

This, then, is one of the key reasons as to why your gut health plays a critical role in your total health. A properly functioning gut, from your mouth to your butt, is what helps your body meet its basic physiological needs in the first place.

If your digestive process, immune system, hormones, mental health, and metabolism are all working *optimally*, there's a good chance that your gut health is working optimally. However, if you have many of the annoying ailments I've mentioned already, there's a good chance that your gut health, which is your body's foundation, has something to do with it. Like a home built on a shaky foundation, if your gut health foundation is shaky, your home (your body) is most likely not as strong as it could be.

If your gut health is contributing to these ailments, and you are perpetually unwell or not at your best, then it is highly unlikely that you will be motivated to move up the hierarchy. After all, it's hard for you to take a step forward toward your goals when you are curled up on the sofa in pain. It's hard to focus on finding motivation when all you are looking for is the toilet.

The list of conditions associated with poor gut health is huge and with a far greater scope than you may realize. Below are some of the common conditions associated with poor gut health:

- ADD/ADHD
- Allergies (seasonal, food)
- Alzheimer's disease
- Anorexia
- Anxiety or depression
- Autism
- Autoimmune disease
- Binge-eating disorder
- Brain fog
- Bulimia
- Candida
- Cancer
- Chronic fatigue
- Colds and flu
- Depression
- Diarrhea
- Diabetes and blood sugar imbalance (hyper/hypoglycemia)
- Endometriosis
- Erectile dysfunction
- Fibromyalgia
- Gallbladder attacks
- Gout
- Headaches
- Heartburn (gastroesophageal reflux disease or GERD)
- High cholesterol and heart disease
- Hormone imbalance (PMS, PCOS, infertility, amenorrhea)
- Irritable bowel syndrome and IBD (Crohn's, colitis)
- Infertility
- Insomnia
- Joint pain
- Loose watery stools
- Low libido
- Lyme disease and co-infections
- Mast Cell Activation Syndrome

- Malabsorption/nutrient deficiency
- Mold illness
- Mood swings
- Muscle pain
- Obesity
- Obsessive Compulsive Disorder
- Osteoporosis and osteopenia
- PCOS
- Personality Disorders
- PMS/PMDD
- Rheumatoid arthritis
- Sinus infections
- Small intestinal bacterial overgrowth (SIBO)
- Skin problems (acne, eczema, rosacea)
- Stuffy nose
- Thyroid disease
- Unintentional weight gain or loss
- Urinary Tract Infections (UTI)
- Yeast infections

Without a healthy gut, we do not absorb the nutrients that feed our brain and every cellular function of our body, and without a well-nourished heart, brain, thyroid, liver, muscles, bones, and beyond, we cannot work our nine-to-five (without a big boost from coffee or sugar), engage in meaningful conversation and relationships, focus on studying or learning, or achieve our wildest dreams. Our energy tanks deplete, our immune system goes down, our hormones poop out, our liver and detox pathways get clogged, our intestines can't properly digest, and our brain's neurotransmitters stop firing correctly.

In short: all disease arises from *dis-ease* in your body, in the second brain, and in your life.

## UNDERSTANDING HOW IDEAL DIGESTION WORKS

If you want to figure out how to optimize your gut, you first need to know how ideal digestion and gut health *should* work in the first place.

Your gut has three primary functions:

- **1) It breaks down the food you eat into nutrients**, which are then absorbed to provide you with energy and nourishment for life, growth, and repair;

- **2) It is responsible for the foundation of your immune system,** housing the majority of your immune cells, metabolizing antioxidants and nutrients to boost immune function, and working closely with your liver to protect you from foreign invaders, like viruses and toxin;
- **3) It is the "conductor" for every bodily process,** containing trillions of gut bacteria, yeasts, and fungi that act like the orchestra for brain function and thoughts. There are more of these microorganisms in your gut than there are cells in your body, and they serve as the primary orchestrators for practically every bodily process, including thyroid function, energy production, hormone balance, metabolism, fitness performance, sleep quality, blood pressure, memory, and so much more.

To do these jobs effectively and *prevent* disease, we want our digestive anatomy and physiology, our gut structure and functions, in tip-top shape.

Here's a biology class refresher:

Your gastrointestinal tract is a thick hollow tube of cells, tissues, blood vessels, and fat that consists of several parts, including your

- Brain;
- Mouth (teeth, salivary glands);
- Pharynx (throat);
- Esophagus (tube down to your stomach);
- Stomach;
- Accessory organs that assist the GI tract, like the liver, gallbladder, and pancreas;
- Small Intestine;
- Large intestine (colon);
- Anus;
- Microbiota: gut bacteria, yeasts, fungi, protozoa (parasites);

The process of digestion happens from north to south—starting up top with the thoughts in your brain (planning to eat and food preparation) and ending down low with the anus (your stool). The entire process can take anywhere from 12–72 hours. Ideally, the goal is a solid 24 hours for one meal.

Any health issues we experience throughout our lives, from strep throat and the flu to headaches and acne, directly reflect what is going on inside our gut (even if we don't feel gassy or bloated).

## IDEAL DIGESTION

Here's a play-by-play of how ideal digestion works:

### *STEP 1: THINK ABOUT FOOD IN YOUR BRAIN*

In step one, food is on the brain. You are planning, thinking about, salivating, and/or obsessing over food. Historically, our ancestors intuitively thought about food when they were hungry and foraged, hunted, and ate to meet their needs. Today, since food is more readily available at the punch of a button, a call of GrubHub, or a stroll to our pantry, ancestral hunger signals have also become more complex, often involving not only *stomach* or *cellular* hunger cues but five other types of hunger as well, including:

- Mouth hunger (hunger when we taste food);
- Eye hunger (hunger when we see food);
- Nose hunger (hunger when we smell food);
- Heart hunger (emotional hunger);
- Mind hunger (hunger from thinking about food);

### *STEP 2: CHEW YOUR FOOD.*

Teeth, through chewing, or mastication, make food easier to swallow. Salivary glands produce enzymes to digest carbohydrates (amylase) and fats (lingual lipase), as well as to spark an immune response to fight foreign invaders and pathogenic bacteria.

*Fun Fact: There are genetic differences in salivary amylase and lingual lipase enzyme production between people, and this is one of the reasons why carbohydrate and fat tolerance varies among individuals (that is, some people digest carbs or fats better than others and why some people feel better with more carbs or more fats in their diet).*

## *STEP 3:* SWALLOW YOUR FOOD.

*Gulp!* Food passes through the pharynx and esophagus—functioning as a transport system between the mouth and the stomach.

## *STEP 4:* FOOD STIMULATES STOMACH ACID & CHYME PRODUCTION.

The stomach is a pit stop, where food remains for 1–2 hours, undergoing a chemistry experiment in your gut as stomach acid and digestive enzymes break food down into chyme. This sludge-like substance consists of food mixed with stomach acid and enzymes, which can pass into the small intestine for protein digestion.

## *STEP 5:* NUTRIENT ABSORPTION & UTILIZATION IN THE SMALL INTESTINE.

The small intestine is an 18-foot-long organ (about the size of three twin mattresses spread out end-to-end). The small intestine contains tons of intestinal microvilli that help absorb nutrients. It is where the majority of digestion and nutrient absorption occurs, for around 6–8 hours. If you feel bloated, constipated, tired, brain foggy, or gassy approximately 2–6 hours after eating, this is an indication that gut problems like small intestinal bacterial overgrowth, fungal overgrowth, and leaky gut may be present.

## *STEP 6:* THE ACCESSORY ORGANS ALSO HELP BREAK DOWN NUTRIENTS AND PATHOGENS.

The liver, gallbladder, and pancreas are called your "accessory organs" and are responsible for creating and signaling digestive enzymes that assist the small intestine with digestion, as well as working to cleanse wastes and toxins.

The *liver* is your body's detox and nutrient-processing factory. *All* nutrients and toxins we eat, inhale, or put on our skin must first pass through the liver to be filtered before traveling anywhere else in the body. It is the liver that decides what to keep and what to get rid of.

The *gallbladder* is the liver's "assistant" organ, like Batman and Robin. Your gallbladder is essential for forming healthy bowel movements, keeping your liver clear of congestion, pumping out toxins in bile, digesting fats, and preventing bloating, constipation, and bacterial or fungal overgrowth.

The *pancreas* is a small organ behind the stomach that creates the majority of enzymes, specializing in plant fibers and starches/carb digestion. Your pancreas also regulates insulin levels for more energy and balanced blood sugar. Considering that nearly 90 percent of people have blood sugar issues, the pancreas has something to do with this.

## *STEP 7:* ***FOOD GETS A FINAL "CLEAN SWEEP" IN THE LARGE INTESTINE (COLON).***

The colon is the master recycler, where all undigested food and fiber pass for a final clean sweep before exiting the body. It also gathers undigested leftovers and indigestible fibers to form your stool. The large intestine is where the vast majority (90 percent) of your gut bacteria *should* reside (both healthy and unhealthy). Ironically, the large intestine is much smaller than the small intestine at about four and a half feet.

## *STEP 8:* ***KICK IT OUT THE BUTT.***

Out the back door! *Ideally,* 19–24 hours after eating a meal, any unnecessary waste exits through the anus in a well-formed, C or S-shaped, softened poo.

The same thing goes for your immune cells, housed in your gut-tissue fluids (also known as GALT—gut-associated lymphatic tissue) and your gut bacteria. If your gut-tissue fluids or gut bacteria are exposed to lots of stressors, and your digestive system is not in excellent shape, then systemic inflammation and suppression or over-activation of your immune system are inevitable. In this case, you don't necessarily have a leaky gut, as many blogosphere health experts may claim, but you certainly have an inflamed gut and/or disrupted gut microbiota.

# CHAPTER 3:
# GUT BACTERIA: YOUR SECRET WEAPONS

Let's chat about your gut bacteria for a moment—consider gut bacteria as your body's secret weapons for total health and body balance. Also, keep in mind that life itself does not exist without bacteria.

Although the word "bacteria" may sound gross or paint images in your mind of the squiggly prokaryotes in your Ninth Grade Biology textbook, consider that you would not exist without them.

You are one of the most densely populated microbial habitats known on earth—five pounds of you represents nearly 100 trillion bacteria—the same amount as cells in the human body and more than the 250 billion stars in the sky.

Contrary to popular belief, gut microbes are friends. Not foes. Ever take antibiotics, sterilize your hands with antimicrobial soap or sanitizer, or use Lysol and Clorox to clean your kitchen countertops?

*Duh. Doesn't everyone?* Unfortunately, we've been misinformed about "germs" our entire life—something called the "germ theory." This theory states that there are fixed, external germs or bacteria which invade the body and are the direct cause of disease. If you truly want to get well, you need to kill whatever germ made you sick and do whatever possible to make "sure" that you never allow a microbe to enter your body in the first place.

With this theory came Western medicine and its tools and technologies to eradicate unfriendly microbes through drugs, surgery, radiation, and chemotherapy.

Interestingly, before the inventor of this theory, Louis Pasteur, died, he retracted his conclusions, saying that gut microbes are friends, not foes, and that our environment and lifestyle influence our health more than bacteria. However, it was too late; the scientific community started already marching on his initial idea, and ever since, modern medicine has been based on this model: *viruses and bacteria cause disease.*

That said, there are two sides to every story.

Most of the bacteria living inside us are *not* bad. Instead, one bacteria and other bacteria can influence entire populations of bacteria together—which is why bacterial balance and diversity are also important.

In fact, in most humans, approximately 1 percent of bacteria are pathogenic strains. The other 99 percent of bacteria living inside us are actually the good guys (like many of the strains found in probiotics)—benefiting the host, as long as they are not overgrown. For example, some gut bacteria like Clostridia can benefit the host by turning dietary fiber into short-chain fatty acids (SCFAs), killing off toxins, and providing a hospitable environment for bacteria to live peacefully. However, if you get an overgrowth of Clostridia, as in the case of a disease called *Clostridium difficile* (*C. diff*), then the commensal can quickly turn pathogenic, causing a diarrhea nightmare.

Additionally, the bacteria in your gut all have different functions. Some metabolize hormones to an active state—like estrogen for fertility, thyroid hormone for energy, or Vitamin D for immunity. Some digest carbs better, whereas others break down fats or proteins; others detox toxins in the water you drink from a plastic water bottle just like the liver does. Hence why diversity is also essential.

*The bottom line: good gut health (and better health overall) is all about the balance and diversity of bacteria species.*

Most people just think about their stomach or GI tract when they hear the word "microbiome." However, your microbiome—the organisms living inside you—goes beyond your stomach. You have various microbiomes for your skin, liver, reproductive glands, mouth, heart, lungs, brain—all of you.

Bacteria—especially healthy bacteria—in each of these regions are the worker bees for various bodily functions, extracting the Omega 3 fatty acids from your salmon dinner, fighting parabens in your Neutrogena face wash and glyphosate in your breakfast Cheerios, boosting your metabolism when you quit chronic dieting, keeping your bowels regular, and guarding against the common cold and allergies.

This is why what you eat, what you breathe in, what you put on your skin, and what health behaviors you do (or don't do) are so important to health—they impact your gut microbiome for better or worse.

For example, when you eat pepperoni pizza, a salad, or a protein bar, you not only feed your cells, but you also feed the trillions of microorganisms living in your gut. The microbes in your gut help break down food, absorb it, and use it (or misuse it) for all your energy needs and bodily systems (hormones, immune, respiratory, brain, liver detox, skin, and more).

The gut bacteria living inside of us are a direct reflection of what passes through our digestive systems.

## THE GOOD, THE BAD, AND THE MUTUALISTIC

Bacteria are often classified in one of three ways:

1. Good (healthy);
2. Bad (pathogenic);
3. Mutualistic or commensal (neither good nor bad).

Most of the bacteria living inside us are *not* bad, and even the bad bacteria are not necessarily bad if you have plenty of healthy bacteria to counter them. What you'll soon learn in reading this book is that such labels are incorrect, if not, on occasion, dangerous.

The concept of simply labeling one bacteria as being "good" or "beneficial" (like *Lactobacillus probiotics*) and one bacteria as just being "bad" or "pathogenic" (like *E. coli*) is not accurate. Instead, one bacteria and other bacteria can influence entire populations of bacteria together, which is why bacterial diversity is also important.

Although there is no single ideal gut microbiome, as long as our biomes are balanced—meaning not too many bacteria of any one strain and not too few bacteria overall, and enough diversity (variety of species)—then we generally are healthy. The greater the microbiome bacterial diversity, the less likely we are to have inflammatory reactions. We have no need for coffee-required energy, and we experience restorative sleep, clear skin, mental clarity, happy hormones, the ability to tolerate a variety of real foods, and minimal gut symptoms.

How can you tell if you have a healthy biome? Well, the signs below are the signs and the telltale markers of a healthy, balanced biome:

- A feeling of overall wellness and balance;
- Quality sleep;
- Energy (no coffee needed);
- Clear skin;
- Balanced blood sugar (not "hangry" before meals; no strong cravings; regular appetite);
- Cognitive or mental clarity;
- A strong immune system;
- Metabolic flexibility;
- Normal thyroid function and hormone balance;
- Ability to eat a variety of real, whole foods (low food intolerances);
- Minimized gut symptoms (minimal bloating, GERD, indigestion, constipation, loose/watery stools, etc.);
- Good detoxification (no mold, heavy metals or gallbladder issues);
- Microbiota diversity; no pathogens.

On the flip side, if our bacteria are off, we call this "dysbiosis"—a fancy word for disrupted gut microbiota.

## DYSBIOSIS DEBRIEF

Dysbiosis, or a disrupted gut microbiota, is one of those *common* but not necessarily *normal* things in our culture—just like consuming Big Macs and Starbucks' Unicorn Frappuccinos are common, but not the healthy, normal foods that the human body is designed to eat.

Dysbiosis affects at least one in two people who have gut-health-related conditions (19), although some experts even say that 74 percent of people live with regular gastrointestinal discomfort, thinking it's "normal" and have never discussed it with their doctor (20). I believe that once you finish this book, you will realize how many areas of your body that your gut health impacts; I think it's safe to say 99.9 percent of people, at least in the US, need to at least think about their gut.

In fact, of all developed nations in the world, the US ranks as Number One with the least diverse microbiomes. We won! We're number one with the most dysbiotic guts in the world (21). Even if you're health-conscious–eating salads from Whole Foods, buying only organic food, crushing a HIIT workout or run every day, and popping probiotics–doing all the right things–you still face *tons* of stressors and environmental factors that affect your gut microbiome, from BPA in plastic water bottles to secondhand smoke, parabens in your shampoo, toxic exhaust from cars on the freeway, mycotoxins, and so much more. We will discuss this in greater detail in the next chapter.

So, what are the signs of dysbiosis?

- Insomnia or poor sleep;
- Pooping every other day (or every few days);
- Frequent loose stools;
- Fatigue;
- Skin problems;
- Sugar or caffeine cravings;
- Brain fog;
- Allergies, autoimmune disease, and poor general immunity;
- Sinus congestion;
- Thyroid and hormone imbalances;
- Food sensitivities and intolerances;
- Environmental sensitivities;
- Chronic joint or muscle pain;
- Inflammation;
- Easily anxious, emotional, or depressed;
- Cavities and dental problems;
- High cholesterol;
- Gut symptoms:
  - *GERD, acid reflux, or heartburn;*
  - *Bloating, gas, cramps, or abdominal pain after eating;*
  - *Nausea;*
  - *Undigested food in stool;*
  - *Yeast overgrowth, or inflammatory gut markers.*

Most people have no idea that they have dysbiosis or a sub-par digestive system—especially since not all gut problems result in chronic TUMS popping or overt gut symptoms, such as bloating, gas, or constipation. Instead, your gut and digestive health affect several other systems, and many of them are systems that have physical symptoms, as highlighted by the list above, that you would never have guessed.

# THE REAL WORLD: GUT CONNECTIONS

Cue the conclusion of Dr. Wennerstrom's boring digestive system lecture. Yet, as you scan the room, the connections finally come to life...

## *REGINA'S METABOLIC MAYHEM*

Beautiful blonde Regina is in the back of the class, snacking on a Kalteen Bar—heavily marketed to "help you lose weight." Lately, she's been doing all the things—paleo, keto, intermittent fasting, celery juice, and macro counting—limiting her carbs to twenty or less per day, and now Kalteen Bars. Yet, nothing has been working. She feels bloated and swollen every morning in her yoga pants, and she can't lose those last ten pounds for the life of her.

## *CASSIE'S CRAVINGS CONUNDRUM*

Speaking of snacking, Cassie, also in the back of the room, is reminded that she is hungry when she hears Regina George peel back the wrapper of her Kalteen Bar. After skipping breakfast, and with it now coming close to lunchtime, all Cassie can think about is food. Just *eight* more minutes. Pizza sticks? Chicken fingers? Onion rings? Ice cream sandwich... What to choose? Maybe all of them? "Hanger" has definitely set in, and her attention is everywhere else but on Biology.

## *IAN'S SKIN BREAKOUTS*

Distracting the entire class up in the front of the classroom is Ian—the 15-year-old performing surgery on the pimples gracing his "pizza face."

Like many teenagers, he's had acne—and "backne"—that he had never been able to solve. He's tried multiple remedies—tanning beds, antibiotics, Accutane, expensive skin care cleansers, red light therapy, and natural face washes. Nothing worked.

Like many Americans, Ian was a product of the "antibiotic-and-Cookie-Crisps-for-breakfast generation" and had his fair share of a youthful history of antibiotic exposures alongside the antibiotics prescribed for his skin condition. There are often more pieces to the skin puzzle beyond your skincare routine.

Little does Ian realize that he has high circulating levels of LPS (lipopolysaccharide), also known as "endotoxins," low Vitamin D, and Intestinal Permeability (aka: "leaky gut"), all exacerbating low-grade inflammation from both food proteins and toxins filtering into his bloodstream.

## *MICHELLE'S HAYWIRE HORMONES*

Michelle can't wait until the class bell rings so she can go change her tampon for the third time today (and it's barely noon). And she needs to make a trip by Nurse Foy's office for Advil. Please give me more Advil! These cramps suck. To make things worse, for some reason, she grabbed her white pants today. *Why?!* She has no idea. #The(PMS)StruggleIsReal.

## *BRIAN NEEDS BRAIN POWER*

Our last friend, Brian, is sitting in the back, *trying* his best to take notes and stay engaged. However, his mind is running like a hamster on a wheel after drinking sugar water at what feels like 120 miles per hour.

*Basketball practice. Small intestines—check. Regina is hot. Mmm...pizza sticks sound good. Regina is hot. Pancreatic enzymes... Oh look, a squirrel!*

"What do you think, Brian?" Dr. Wennerstrom calls on him.

"*Whaaat?* Can you repeat the question?"

The ADD struggle is *also* real.

* * *

These stories are based on hypothetical scenarios, things we all will have seen growing up and can personally relate to. We have all experienced or seen someone experiencing these things. Now, though, I want to take you to some real-world scenarios that I personally have experienced as a clinician. The names have been changed, but the stories have not.

## *CHRISTY'S METABOLIC MAYHEM*

Christy was 42 years old when she came to me feeling "fat, foggy, and fatigued," as she put it.

"I just don't get it. I eat healthily, work out, and drink water," she told me. No matter what she tried, she didn't feel good. Her PMS was a struggle, she woke up with swollen lymph nodes every morning, and she couldn't lose those last ten pounds no matter what she tried. And she'd tried it all: paleo, keto, intermittent fasting, celery juice, and macro counting, even limiting her carbs to twenty grams or less per day.

By the time she saw me, she was eating the same 5–10 high-protein, high-fat foods every day and felt guilty if she even played with the idea of eating a starchy vegetable like butternut squash. She was also taking her own poly-pharmacy of supplements, which included a generic probiotic she found at Target, licorice and cordyceps for more energy, a multivitamin and Vitamin-B complex, a detox formula, and a thyroid glandular (because she heard that supporting the thyroid is good for metabolism). However, none of it was working.

In response to her highly negative mindset, exasperated by the lack of real results, I encouraged her to take a step back to review and assess the positives, negatives, and the "I don't know" variables that made her feel better. Through doing this, we identified just how exhausting keeping track of this routine must have been, not to mention expensive, so we cut out unnecessary supplements, and the initial workup included:

- Keeping a three-day food and poo log;
- Comprehensive stool analysis;
- A DUTCH cortisol hormone test;
- A blood sugar tracking log, and;
- A therapeutic supplement trial of stomach acid support (apple cider vinegar) and digestive bitters to support her gallbladder to see how her body responded.

Through testing, it emerged that Christy's free cortisol—the hormone that creates stress—levels were off the charts, particularly at night time (when they should be low) after a long day's work, explaining why she had difficulty sleeping for more than 4–5 hours per night, and the reason she felt so tired most days. Ironically, the licorice she had been taking was actually counterproductive—licorice elevates cortisol. Couple this with a candida (yeast) presentation on her stool test, gallbladder congestion preventing complete digestion (especially of fats on a keto diet), and sluggish liver clearance of her hormones thanks to her 14-year history on the birth control pill, and we had some "meat" to work with to begin transforming her body. In as little as two months, Christy went from "fat, foggy, and fatigued" to shedding the need for coffee-based energy, losing five pounds of inflammation, and enjoying seven hours of uninterrupted sleep on most nights.

Your gut dictates your metabolism—how your body breaks food down to use and store energy.

Looking at your gut bacteria, researchers can tell whether you're overweight or lean. For example, both mice and humans that receive gut bacteria transplants from overweight mice or humans gain more weight than subjects transplanted with gut bacteria from normal weight or lean subjects—even when they eat the same diet.

Have you ever wondered why news headlines say that 95 percent of all diets fail? It may be because of what's going on in the gut. One study (3) in obese mice revealed a positive change in their gut microbiota during weight loss; however, after the diet ended and the gut was no longer supported by a healthy diet, the weight lost was quickly regained. The same study also showed that adding antibiotics—known for altering the gut microbiota—further accelerated regained weight.

The *Biggest Loser* study (22) is another perfect example of this. You've probably heard of the show, which is a contest to see how quickly a group of obese people can lose weight. What they don't show you is that when researchers tested the metabolic rates of previous contestants six years following the show, they found that nearly all of the contestants had regained the pounds. On top of that, their metabolism had slowed, and they were burning fewer calories every day than before the show's start.

The key takeaway? Your metabolism and body composition are dependent on more than 1,200 calorie diets and marathon spin classes (and those may actually be counterproductive to a healthy gut in the long run).

## HAYLEE'S DISORDERED EATING

Haylee was a 26-year-old woman with a history of disordered eating. As a teen, she went through a phase of food restriction and over-exercise, followed by college days characterized by weekly binge-purge episodes, especially after a night of drinking. Post-college, she started her first 9–5 desk job and decided that she also wanted to develop new healthy habits with her new work routine. In the spirit of "feeling good," Haylee packed dry leafy green salads for work, prepped chicken and broccoli for dinner, tracked her steps daily, and joined a gym. However, several years into this routine, she hit a wall.

She often obsessed over food and found herself craving foods she knew she "shouldn't" have. Some days were better than others, but not a week went by that she did not find herself in the work break room with her hand in a cookie jar, sneaking a pint of Ben & Jerry's after a tough workout, or driving through the Chick-fil-A drive-thru for a large lemonade, chicken nuggets, and waffle fries.

"I know I shouldn't eat these things, but I get so bored with chicken and broccoli that I just crave the treats!" She explained. On top of feeling defeated by food, she also experienced bloating after most meals and "hanger"—that feeling of hunger and anger if she went too long between meals in the latter half of the day.

One look at her daily lifestyle log revealed that she was significantly undereating, often not eating her first meal most days until noon or 1 p.m., and stacking her 1,200 to 1,400 calories most days within a matter of hours with higher carbohydrate, lower protein meals.

She also did not chew her food enough: an average habit of taking 5–7 bites before each swallow severely impacted her body's absorption abilities. Additionally, her gut motility was highly stressed (HPA axis dysregulation). Her average breath rate during the day was twenty breaths per minute, signaling "freeze" instead of "digest" to her gut motility, resulting in all the bloating, and leptin resistance—inability to feel fullness—was overtly present due to HPA axis dysregulation as well. A SIBO breath test further confirmed a hydrogen-based presentation of bacterial overgrowth in her upper GI tract, supporting her junk food cravings and sweet tooth; her comprehensive hormone analysis revealed high metabolized cortisol with sharp declines at sugar-craving times during the day (mid-afternoon and late evening).

Unlike other trainers, nutritionists, therapists, and doctors who had told her to "go keto," "go on a sugar cleanse," "try harder," take an anxiety pill, or "get her thyroid checked," by instead looking closely at the nature of her gut-brain axis Haylee was able to connect many of the dots between her gut and her binging habits.

Have you ever craved food that you know makes you feel bad but ate it anyway? Nearly 100 percent of women and 70 percent of men report regularly experiencing cravings for certain foods, often foods that don't make them feel good (23).

This craving is due to your gut microbes telling your brain what foods your body "needs" by suppressing or increasing cravings.

Since gut bacteria feed on whatever their host animal eats, if you have disrupted digestion or nutrient malabsorption, this creates an imbalanced gut rich in bacteria that tell your brain to feed them more foods that help them thrive and ferment. These craving signals are sent to your brain through the "gut-brain" axis—the direct telephone line for communication between the gut and the brain. Your gut-brain axis is constantly communicating, and when it comes to food cravings, signals in your brain and gut allow them to talk to each other. Inflammation in your gut or brain tends to make you crave and want foods that meet your needs for instant gratification. It's no wonder, then, that mental health conditions like anxiety, ADHD/ADD, and depression have been associated with both dysbiosis *and* an increased likelihood of eating unhealthy foods (24, 25).

Different bacteria prefer different food sources (26). While most gut bugs are generalists able to thrive on a variety of substrates, they usually prefer one particular food group over another based on the amount of energy they save during the process of digestion. For example, *Lactobacilli* tend to like sugars and starches, *Prevotella* love carbs, *Bacteroidetes* prefer fats, *Clostridium* enjoys proteins, and *Bifidobacteria* take the lead when it comes to fermenting fiber. These bacteria require a steady intake of their preferred food types to grow and reproduce.

Likewise, certain bacteria *don't* like specific food types, explaining why some kids and adults strongly despise vegetables like Brussels sprouts and broccoli—remember those Supertasters I mentioned earlier? Taste perceptions and preferences are governed by gut bacteria. Supertasters have a completely different microbial profile than those with less intense taste buds—specifically for bitter and astringent compounds (such as caffeine, teas, spices, vegetables, and fruits) and flavorings such as salt, sugar, and acid. This also explains why older adults tend to tolerate and gravitate towards foods with stronger flavors (sour, spicy) and sweets as they age: their gut bacteria change (27–29).

Certain foods and food products themselves also contain chemicals that alter not only our gut microbiome but also the neurotransmitters produced by our gut microbiome. For example, cheese contains casein and casein fragments called casomorphins, a casein-derived, morphine-like compound with opiate (drug-like) molecules built in. When consumed, these fragments attach to the same brain receptors to which heroin and other narcotics attach. Our brain's reward center releases serotonin and dopamine when we eat salty foods like cheese to encourage us to eat more. The same thing happens with foods like Doritos, French fries, sugar, and even "diet" foods like diet soda, sugar-free ice cream, processed bars, and any other food you feel like you have to have every day. Patients with anorexia are reported to have compulsive food behaviors (30, 31), like how I consumed bland frozen turkey burgers, over-steamed broccoli, and Crystal Light every day for years. Researchers speculate that women with anorexia, who usually have significant insufficiency dysbiosis (low diversity of gut bacteria), respond to this phenomenon (31).

## *SETH'S STORY*

Seth was a healthy guy—at least most people thought so. He was a top-performing CEO of a successful startup at the young age of 32. He also had a strong interest in bio-hacking, using blue blocker glasses at night, infrared saunas regularly, and sleeping in a pitch-black 68-degree room for optimal sleep hygiene.

On top of this, he was active and fit. Seth performed CrossFit four to five days per week and was training for a Spartan Race. He followed a ketogenic diet: Low on carbs but high on quality fats and organic proteins. Breakfast was bulletproof coffee with a heaping scoop of collagen, butter, and MCT oil. Lunch was bone broth and a salad with chicken or fish, and dinner was meat and veggies drizzled with olive oil. His only "downfall" was the occasional grass-fed cheese, Keto snack bars if he was on the go, and his love of beer on the weekends—a few with his buddies over football or at the bar. Oh yes, and he had acne, or rather, "backne," that he had never been able to solve. This was what brought Seth to me. He'd tried everything, all of the stuff Ian, whom I referenced earlier, had tried, but like Ian, nothing had worked.

Lo and behold, Seth had high circulating levels of LPS detected on an Intestinal Permeability screening, creating a condition called "metabolic endotoxemia"—persistent, low-grade inflammation from both food proteins and toxins filtering into his bloodstream. Additionally, his stool test revealed a low growth of beneficial bacteria and the detection of some opportunistic flora often found on the skin and in the GI tract that causes infections in acne patients, particularly those who have undergone long-term antibiotic therapy. On top of Seth's GI test findings, we also discovered he had low Vitamin D, B-Vitamin deficiency (pernicious anemia), and elevated thyroid antibodies, impairing his immune function and skin repair abilities.

Seventy to eighty percent of your immune system is produced and housed in your gut, specifically T cells, which are critical for fighting pathogens, disease, and acne (fun fact: your skin is your largest immune organ). The healthier your gut, the stronger your immune system, and the less likely you are to get disease or experience imbalances. If immune imbalances *do* arise, like allergies, a cold or flu, nausea, headaches, fatigue, and more, boosting and building up your gut will result in a faster bounce back. End of story.

Unfortunately, a vast majority of people do not have a strong immune system, pointing to the fact that many of us do not have a strong GI system. Nearly one in three Americans suffer from allergies, and one in five has an autoimmune disease—one of the fastest-growing chronic diseases to date.

Common colds are the main reason that children miss school and adults miss work, with most adults catching two to three colds per year, and children, eight to ten. Furthermore, one out of two adults experiences adult acne, which, believe it or not, is the result of your skin being part of your immune system (25-30).

That said, occasional illness is a part of life. In fact, it can actually be a good thing, a sign that your immune system is activated and can work. People who *never* get sick may have the opposite problem—no immune cells to mount an immune response at all. What matters is your body's ability to bounce back instead of staying sick. People with strong immune systems, better digestion, and a healthier gut generally will bounce back from sinus congestion or a sore throat in a couple of days. In contrast, people with weaker immune systems find their healing time dragging on, feel a general sense of fatigue, or continue to get sick repetitively.

## MICHELLE'S THYROID NIGHTMARE

Michelle came to me as a 44-year-old female recently diagnosed with Hashimoto's disease—an autoimmune disease of the thyroid—after years of reportedly not feeling like herself. Thankfully, she found a practitioner who finally asked if she had had her thyroid antibodies checked. She never had. Her TPO antibodies (an autoimmune thyroid marker) were off the charts at 356, where the normal is under 35, her Vitamin D was at 19, and her B vitamins were in the low 200s.

She came to me after having been told she'd soon need to start taking a steroid drug to calm her inflammation and that she would be on thyroid medication for the rest of her life, as the doctor hypothesized that her thyroid levels would most likely worsen.

"Is there anything else I can do?" she asked me in my office, tears filling her eyes. I suggested we do a bit more digging to help figure out what had triggered her Hashimoto's in the first place.

Upon initial workup and further examination, we discovered that Michelle had been living in a moldy rental home for the past three years, about the same timeline she attributed to worsening her symptoms—low energy, IBS, painful periods, and brain fog. Prior to her move into the home, she also had gone on a trip to Turkey and remembered one bad night of food poisoning. From then on, she said her poor health, low energy, and autoimmune symptoms really began to arise.

A mycotoxin urine test revealed elevated ochratoxins, aspergillus species, and mild yeast overgrowth. Michelle also had a parasite, along with low secretory IgA (chronic immune marker in the gut). Despite being low in her Vitamin D and B counts, she also presented with high iron markers (iron overload), suggesting inflammation and a further contributor to the autoimmune attack of her thyroid.

"How come no one ever told me any of this?" she asked.

Hormone health goes hand-in-hand with the functioning of your gut.

Underlying gut stress is correlated with estrogen and testosterone imbalances primarily because normal hormone production is altered.

For example, in the case of estrogen dominance, gut bacteria that metabolize estrogens can produce an enzyme (beta-glucuronidase) that activates the release of *extra* estrogen inside your gut. This re-activated estrogen then re-enters your body and can cause high estrogen symptoms, including PMS and period "problems," menopausal hot flashes, mood swings, and "man boobs." Long-term birth control use (elevated estrogens) is also associated with increased bacterial overgrowth, like SIBO, dysbiosis, and "leaky gut." A Harvard study linked the use of birth control to a 300 percent increase in risk for Crohn's disease (33). Contraceptives, including the pill, IUDs, and the NuvaRing, have also been linked to both long-term hormonal imbalances and gut issues.

As for women with low estrogen who experience infertility or secondary amenorrhea (period loss), studies commonly show significant differences in gut bacteria (dysbiosis), as well as decreased gut motility with symptoms of constipation, IBS, and bloating.

On the testosterone front, metabolic endotoxemia (leaky gut) decreases the body's natural production of testosterone—an androgen hormone needed in both men and women, in the right amounts, for libido, muscle and bone growth, metabolism, energy, mood, and cognitive function. Several animal and human studies show significant positive improvements in testosterone when subjects are administered probiotics and friendly gut bugs are activated.

Lastly, we can't talk about your hormones and gut health without talking about the thyroid. Your thyroid is a vital, butterfly-shaped hormone gland located in your throat that acts as your metabolic mothership, regulating body temperature regulation, heart rate, and blood pressure, calorie and nutrient use, body weight and metabolism, immune system function, digestion, and sex hormone production. Approximately 60 to 70 percent of the thyroid hormone is converted in the gut and liver. If your gut is *unable* to make that conversion, thyroid dysfunction may occur.

That was Michelle's case.

## *NICK'S DEPRESSED GUT*

When I met Nick, he was 55 years old. He had struggled with depression and anxiety for as long as he could remember.

"I will probably always be this way—I don't know any different," he told me.

He clearly did not see a way out. Between losing his job of 26 years the previous spring, being verbally abused by his parents growing up, struggling with parenting his rebellious young adult daughter, and not knowing what to do next in his career, he was constantly at war with himself and the negative thoughts, emotions, and feeling of being overwhelmed that filled his head on a daily basis.

Nick was looking to explore anything that may help him feel better. Between us, we discovered that Nick's gut health and lifestyle did not support a healthier brain space. His daily vegan diet consisting of energy bars, black bean burgers, quinoa bowls, and fruit left him significantly deficient in nutrients, particularly in the essential B vitamins, zinc, magnesium, and iron. He also had an extensive history of lowered immunity paired with antibiotic exposure—from strep throat to sinus infections and allergies; to a history of being treated with medication for ADHD as a kid; and most recently being diagnosed with Crohn's disease, pointing to a leaky gut and dysbiosis.

"I've done everything—medications, therapy, groups, yoga, positive thinking, a support dog—but nothing is helping," Nick said at our first appointment. When we did our full assessment and uncovered the following findings, Nick had a better idea of what he was facing:

- Insufficiency dysbiosis (not enough healthy gut bacteria);
- Low metabolized cortisol and high free cortisol (driving the inflammatory cascade inside);
- An *H. pylori* bacterial infection in his gut;
- Low serotonin and melatonin on his neurotransmitter markers from the DUTCH test;
- Low Vitamin D;
- The MTFHR gene revealing poor methylation;
- Food intolerance to dairy and difficulty digesting FODMAPS, given his gut conditions.

Gut bacteria control your thoughts. Rember, you have more than 500 million neurons inside your gut—brain cells that talk directly to the brain. A healthy, happy gut sends happy thoughts, contributing to less brain inflammation and distraction overall.

*Gut stress affects brain stress.* Have you ever felt constipated or bloated, and all you could think about was the discomfort in your gut? Sort of like a baby who has to do the "doo"—they fuss, cry, and get all wound up until, voila, the golden poo! Or perhaps you've eaten a glazed chocolate donut, artificially sweetened diet soda, or McDonald's French fries and felt a euphoric brain fog afterward—unable to concentrate or think straight. Do you get afternoon energy crashes and headaches every day at 3 p.m. due to poor digestion and hypoglycemia? Caffeine and sugar are all you can keep your mind on?

*Brain stress equally affects gut stress.* For example, the simple thought of eating your mom's warm, homemade chocolate chip cookies can release the stomach's juices before food gets there. Emotional distress over a bad breakup or stress at work can leave your stomach tied up in knots—not hungry or else insatiably hungry, unable to get your emotional fill through food. And the very idea of public speaking or singing on stage in a roomful of strangers can make your stomach feel like it's floating away.

I wish I could say these stories were fiction—made-up stories. They are not. Different symptoms. Different stories. One similar underlying root cause: Gut and digestive imbalance.

Some people think that our genes are the reason we get certain diseases, meaning that they just have to settle for their slow metabolism, daily headaches, seasonal allergies, or bad sleep. However, your genes are not your destiny—they're responsible for only 5-10 percent of all health outcomes. The other 90-95 percent of how you feel? You have your gut biome balance and your multiple gut-axises to thank for that. (45).

Health is an inside job. When you optimize your gut, you optimize your total health.

## REFERENCES


1. A.K. Abbas, A.H.H. Lichtman, S. Pillai, Cellular and Molecular Immunology E-Book, Elsevier Health Sciences, 2017.
2. Froehlich, Eleonore & Wahl, Richard. (2019). Microbiota and Thyroid Interaction in Health and Disease. Trends in Endocrinology & Metabolism. 30. 10.1016/j.tem.2019.05.008.
3. Baker, James & Al-Nakkash, Layla & Herbst-Kralovetz, Melissa. (2017). Estrogen–Gut Microbiome Axis: Physiological and Clinical Implications. Maturitas. 103. 10.1016/j.maturitas.2017.06.025.
4. Tremellen, K., McPhee, N., Pearce, K., Benson, S., Schedlowski, M., & Engler, H. (2018). Endotoxin-initiated inflammation reduces testosterone production in men of reproductive age. *American journal of physiology. Endocrinology and metabolism*, *314*(3), E206–E213. doi:10.1152/ajpendo.00279.2017

5. Martin, C. R., Osadchiy, V., Kalani, A., & Mayer, E. A. (2018). The Brain-Gut-Microbiome Axis. *Cellular and molecular gastroenterology and hepatology*, 6(2), 133–148. doi:10.1016/j.jcmgh.2018.04.003

6. Thomas C. Fung, Helen E. Vuong, Cristopher D. G. Luna, Geoffrey N. Pronovost, Antoniya A. Aleksandrova, Noah G. Riley, Anastasia Vavilina, Julianne McGinn, Tomiko Rendon, Lucy R. Forrest, Elaine Y. Hsiao. Intestinal serotonin and fluoxetine exposure modulate bacterial colonization in the gut. *Nature Microbiology*, 2019; DOI: 10.1038/s41564-019-0540-4

7. Lyte M. (2013). Microbial endocrinology in the microbiome-gut-brain axis: how bacterial production and utilization of neurochemicals influence behavior. *PLoS pathogens*, 9(11), e1003726. doi:10.1371/journal.ppat.1003726

8. Serge Rezzi, Ziad Ramadan, François-Pierre J. Martin, Laurent B. Fay, Peter van Bladeren, John C. Lindon, Jeremy K. Nicholson, and, and Sunil Kochhar. (2007) Human Metabolic Phenotypes Link Directly to Specific Dietary Preferences in Healthy Individuals. Journal of Proteome Research. 6 (11), 4469-4477. DOI: 10.1021/pr070431h

9. Kalliomäki, Marko & Collado, Maria Carmen & Salminen, Seppo & Isolauri, Erika. (2008). Early difference in fecal microbiota composition in children may predict overweight. The American journal of clinical nutrition. 87. 534-8. 10.1093/ajcn/87.3.534.

10. Depommier C, Everard A, Druart C, *et al.* Supplementation with Akkermansia muciniphila in overweight and obese human volunteers: a proof-of-concept exploratory study. Nat Med. 2019. doi: 10.1038/s41591-019-0495-2.

11. Centers for Disease Control. 2019. Chronic Diseases in America. https://www.cdc.gov/chronicdisease/resources/infographic/chronic-diseases.htm

12. Kotzampassi, Katerina. (2013). Bacteria and Obesity: The Proportion Makes the Difference. Surgery: Current Research. 03. 10.4172/2161-1076.1000152.

13. Davis C. D. (2016). The Gut Microbiome and Its Role in Obesity. *Nutrition today*, *51*(4), 167–174. doi:10.1097/NT.0000000000000167

14. Fothergill, E., Guo, J., Howard, L., Kerns, J. C., Knuth, N. D., Brychta, R., ... Hall, K. D. (2016). Persistent metabolic adaptation 6 years after "The Biggest Loser" competition. *Obesity (Silver Spring, Md.), 24*(8), 1612–1619. doi:10.1002/oby.21538

15. Weingarten, Harvey & Elston, Dawn. (1992). Food cravings in a college population. Appetite. 17. 167-75. 10.1016/0195-6663(91)90019-O.

16. Rogers, G. B., Keating, D. J., Young, R. L., Wong, M. L., Licinio, J., & Wesselingh, S. (2016). From gut dysbiosis to altered brain function and mental illness: mechanisms and pathways. *Molecular psychiatry, 21*(6), 738–748. doi:10.1038/mp.2016.50

17. Jim E. Banta, Gina Segovia-Siapco, Christine Betty Crocker, Danielle Montoya, Noara Alhusseini. Mental health status and dietary intake among California adults: a population-based survey. *International Journal of Food Sciences and Nutrition,* 2019; 1 DOI: 10.1080/09637486.2019.1570085

18. Wu, G. D., Chen, J., Hoffmann, C., Bittinger, K., Chen, Y. Y., Keilbaugh, S. A., ... Lewis, J. D. (2011). Linking long-term dietary patterns with gut microbial enterotypes. *Science (New York, N.Y.), 334*(6052), 105–108. doi:10.1126/science.1208344

19. Cattaneo, Camilla & Gargari, Giorgio & Koirala, Ranjan & Laureati, M. & Riso, Patrizia & Guglielmetti, Simone & Pagliarini, Ella. (2019). New insights into the relationship between taste perception and oral microbiota composition. Scientific Reports. 9. 3549. 10.1038/s41598-019-40374-3.

20. Sergi, Giuseppe & Bano, Giulia & Pizzato, Simona & Veronese, Nicola & Manzato, Enzo. (2016). Taste Loss in the Elderly: Possible Implications for Dietary Habits. Critical reviews in food science and nutrition. 57. 10.1080/10408398.2016.1160208.

21. Nagpal, R., Mainali, R., Ahmadi, S., Wang, S., Singh, R., Kavanagh, K., ... Yadav, H. (2018). Gut microbiome and aging: Physiological and mechanistic insights. *Nutrition and healthy aging, 4*(4), 267–285. doi:10.3233/NHA-170030

22. Glenny, E. M., Bulik-Sullivan, E. C., Tang, Q., Bulik, C. M., & Carroll, I. M. (2017). Eating Disorders and the Intestinal Microbiota: Mechanisms of Energy Homeostasis and Behavioral Influence. *Current psychiatry reports, 19*(8), 51. doi:10.1007/s11920-017-0797-3

23. Garcia-Burgos, D., Maglieri, S., Vögele, C., & Munsch, S. (2018). How Does Food Taste in Anorexia and Bulimia Nervosa? A Protocol for a Quasi-Experimental, Cross-Sectional Design to Investigate Taste Aversion or Increased Hedonic Valence of Food in Eating Disorders. *Frontiers in psychology, 9*, 264. doi:10.3389/fpsyg.2018.00264

24. Seitz, J., Belheouane, M., Schulz, N., Dempfle, A., Baines, J. F., & Herpertz-Dahlmann, B. (2019). The Impact of Starvation on the Microbiome and Gut-Brain Interaction in Anorexia Nervosa. *Frontiers in endocrinology, 10*, 41. doi:10.3389/fendo.2019.00041

25. American Academy of Allergy, Asthma & Immunology. 2018. Allergy Statistics. https://www.aaaai.org/about-aaaai/newsroom/allergy-statistics

26. C Burch, Rebecca & Loder, Stephen & Loder, Elizabeth & Smitherman, Todd. (2015). The Prevalence and Burden of Migraine and Severe Headache in the United States: Updated Statistics From Government Health Surveillance Studies. Headache. 55. 21-34. 10.1111/head.12482.

27. Centers for Disease Control. 2018. Common Colds: Protect Yourself and Others. https://www.cdc.gov/features/rhinoviruses/index.html

28. American Autoimmune Related Diseases Association, Inc. 2017. How many Americans have an autoimmune disease? https://www.aarda.org/knowledge-base/many-americans-autoimmune-disease/

29. Zeichner, J. A., Baldwin, H. E., Cook-Bolden, F. E., Eichenfield, L. F., Fallon-Friedlander, S., & Rodriguez, D. A. (2017). Emerging Issues in Adult Female Acne. *The Journal of clinical and aesthetic dermatology, 10*(1), 37–46.

30. Rocha, M. A., & Bagatin, E. (2018). Adult-onset acne: prevalence, impact, and management challenges. *Clinical, cosmetic and investigational dermatology, 11*, 59–69. doi:10.2147/CCID.S137794

31. Sharp, S. P., Avram, D., Stain, S. C., & Lee, E. C. (2017). Local and systemic Th17 immune response associated with advanced stage colon cancer. *The Journal of surgical research, 208*, 180–186. doi:10.1016/j.jss.2016.09.038

32. Perez-Munoz, Maria & Bergstrom, Kirk & Peng, Vincent & Schmaltz, Robert & Jimenez-Cardona, Roberto & Marsteller, Nathan & McGee, Sam & Clavel, Thomas & Ley, Ruth & Xia, Lijun & Peterson, Daniel. (2014). Discordance between changes in the gut microbiota and pathogenicity in a mouse model of spontaneous colitis. Gut microbes. 5. 10.4161/gmic.28622.

33. Khalili H. (2016). Risk of Inflammatory Bowel Disease with Oral Contraceptives and Menopausal Hormone Therapy: Current Evidence and Future Directions. *Drug safety, 39*(3), 193–197. doi:10.1007/s40264-015-0372-y

34. Poutahidis, T., Springer, A., Levkovich, T., Qi, P., Varian, B. J., Lakritz, J. R., ... Erdman, S. E. (2014). Probiotic microbes sustain youthful serum testosterone levels and testicular size in aging mice. *PloS one, 9*(1), e84877. doi:10.1371/journal.pone.0084877

35. Matos, J. F., Americo, M. F., Sinzato, Y. K., Volpato, G. T., Corá, L. A., Calabresi, M. F., Oliveira, R. B., Damasceno, D. C., ... Miranda, J. R. (2016). Role of sex hormones in gastrointestinal motility in pregnant and non-pregnant rats. *World journal of gastroenterology, 22*(25), 5761-8.

36. Everson, Gregory. (1993). Gastrointestinal motility in pregnancy. Gastroenterology clinics of North America. 21. 751-76.

37. Ashish, Badiye & Neeti, Kapoor & Himanshu, Khajuria. (2013). Copper Toxicity: A Comprehensive Study. Journal of Recent Sciences. 2. 58-67.

38. Anette Rickenlund, Maria J. Eriksson, Karin Schenck-Gustafsson, Angelica Lindén Hirschberg, Amenorrhea in Female Athletes Is Associated with Endothelial Dysfunction and Unfavorable Lipid Profile, *The Journal of Clinical Endocrinology & Metabolism*, Volume 90, Issue 3, 1 March 2005, Pages 1354–1359, https://doi.org/10.1210/jc.2004-1286

39. Tidjani ALou, Maryam & Lagier, Jean-Christophe & Raoult, Didier. (2016). Diet Influence on the Gut Microbiota and Dysbiosis related to Nutritional Disorders. Human Microbiome Journal. 1. 10.1016/j.humic.2016.09.001.

40. Varian, B. J., Poutahidis, T., DiBenedictis, B. T., Levkovich, T., Ibrahim, Y., Didyk, E., ... Erdman, S. E. (2017). Microbial lysate upregulates host oxytocin. *Brain, behavior, and immunity, 61*, 36–49. doi:10.1016/j.bbi.2016.11.002

41. Jamilian, M., Mansury, S., Bahmani, F., Heidar, Z., Amirani, E., & Asemi, Z. (2018). The effects of probiotic and selenium co-supplementation on parameters of mental health, hormonal profiles, and biomarkers of inflammation and oxidative stress in women with polycystic ovary syndrome. *Journal of ovarian research, 11*(1), 80. doi:10.1186/s13048-018-0457-1

42. Karamali, Maryam & Eghbalpour, Sara & Rajabi, Sajad & Jamilian, Mehri & Bahmani, Fereshteh & Tajabadi-Ebrahimi, Maryam & Keneshlou, Fariba & Mirhashemi, Seyyed Mehdi & Chamani, Maryam & Gelougerdi, Sara & Asemi, Zatollah. (2018). Effects of Probiotic Supplementation on Hormonal Profiles, Biomarkers of Inflammation and Oxidative Stress in Women With Polycystic Ovary Syndrome: A Randomized, Double-Blind, Placebo-Controlled Trial. Archives of Iranian Medicine. 21. 1-7.

43. American Thyroid Association. 2019. General Information/Press Room. https://www.thyroid.org/media-main/press-room/

44. Rappaport S. M. (2016). Genetic Factors Are Not the Major Causes of Chronic Diseases. *PloS one, 11*(4), e0154387. doi:10.1371/journal.pone.0154387

45. Fox News. 2015. Survey shows 74 percent of Americans living with GI discomfort. Retrieved from: https://www.foxnews.com/health/survey-shows-74-percent-of-americans-living-with-gi-discomfort

46. Segata N. Gut Microbiome: Westernization and the Disappearance of Intestinal Diversity. *Curr Biol.* 2015;25(14):R611-R613. doi:10.1016/j.cub.2015.05.040

CHAPTER 4:

# THE NUMBER ONE CAUSE OF GUT PROBLEMS

It's the noon lunch rush at Whole Foods Market in downtown Austin, the company's international headquarters.

I was there, setting up "shop" to continue writing this very Chapter.

As I get comfortable, a stranger, we'll call him John, flies in and plops down in the chair next to me with what is likely an 18-dollar cardboard box from the hot bar filled with broccoli, grilled salmon, tofu, squash, and some quinoa-kale-cranberry salad, along with what could be coffee number three of the day. He's wearing a hoodie sweatshirt, Bluetooth earbuds, and a cell phone attached to his hip.

"Tom, I'll call you back, I'm in a time crunch," he says, now whipping his MacBook Pro out of his backpack.

He takes his marks with his right hand on the keyboard, his left hand on his fork and box, and the race begins: Typing and scrolling, *bite* typing and scrolling, *bite* typing and scrolling, *BIG bite*; more typing, more scrolling *Chew* *Chew* *Swallow*.

John is positively shoveling broccoli, salmon, and quinoa in his mouth, straining his neck, and moving his face closer to the screen. He follows this dietary drag race with a swig of coffee, more furious typing, and silencing the buzz on his phone.

Within 15 minutes of sitting down to eat, He is up and at it again. For John, there is simply not enough time in the day. He is always on the move, running to the next place.

## EXHIBIT A: HOW THE GUT GOES BAD.

One word: ***Stress.***

Bad digestion or poor gut health does not happen overnight. Sure, some people are born with genetic mutations or structural imbalances (such as a larger colon or obstructions in their intestinal tract), but the majority of gut health imbalances occur due to stress and imbalance in our gut microbiota (our gut bacteria), causing a domino effect with other aspects of our health.

Further complicating things, many of the stressors to a healthy gut are actually often considered normal—not stressful—in our daily lives.

For John, eating on the go, inadequately chewing his food, eating while glued to a screen, and swigging back yet more coffee was his norm. Just like for others, whose norms might consist of eating Dunkin' Donuts, drinking artificially sweetened diet soda, fighting daily headaches with ibuprofen, undertaking weekly allergy shots, sleeping six hours every night, ordering canola-oil drenched takeout, checking Instagram 42 times daily, and sitting for 12-plus hours every day. Even for those who are "health conscious," their norms may consist of waking up at 4:30 a.m. every morning, running six miles without any rest built in, eating less than twenty carbs and fasting for 16 hours daily, consuming three cups of mycotoxin-free coffee (in order to go Number Two) and simply not listening to their body.

But are these habits *really* normal for humans? Well, not quite.

## EXHIBIT B: HOW THE GUT GOES BAD.

Answer: ***Abnormal lifestyle and nutrition factors.***

Does anything come to mind for you?

My stressful childhood health habits are a perfect example of this—characterized by a steady diet of processed breakfast cereals and Goldfish crackers with a 20-year shelf life, several rounds of antibiotics for my recurring strep throats and ear infections, high-sugar apple juice, orange juice in lieu of water, and popping TUMS like candy: Common things that clearly contributed to gut problems early on.

### *EXAMPLE:* ***CONSTIPATION CALAMITY***

Plop. A small rock-sized nugget, but at least it's something. Another day in Porcelain Paradise (A.K.A Constipation Land).

Even as an 8-year-old, I knew something was up. No matter how much fiber-rich all-bran cereal or prunes I ate, TUMS and Miralax I took, or fluids I drank, my stool and bloating problems didn't go away.

"Some people just get IBS, Lauryn," Dr. Joe said.

No one ever told me my experience was *not* normal—or at least it did not have to be.

You can tell a lot about your gut health simply by looking at your poo—your daily report card. Although everybody poops, not all poop is created equal.

Generally, Golden Poo entails:

- Going 1-2 times per day;
- Well-formed, sausage-like, and C-shaped waste;
- Smooth movements that are easy to pass;
- The feeling of complete elimination, released in 1-3 good chunks;
- No reliance on coffee, laxatives, or other digestive aids.

Only about one out of three Americans pass the Golden Poo test on a daily basis (9)—experiencing instead a variety of stools ranging from hard and cracked to loose and watery, difficult to pass, and everything in between.

# The Golden Poo CHART

What does your *poo* say about you? Check out this chart and see.

Keep a 3 day food & poo log and notice if you see any themes between what you eat and what your poo says about you.

Different types of poo can be attributed to tons of different causes. The key is focusing on the baseline essentials for good digestion, including: chewing your food, stomach acid, digestive enzymes, water with minerals added, a balanced diet, daily movement and quality sleep.

## IDEAL: The Golden Poo:

Happy gut. Dark brown. C or S-shaped. Easy to pass in 1-2 pushes.

**FAKE OUT:** Well formed, BUT reddened or light brown poo: gut inflammation, dysbiosis, low stomach acid, red stools may also indicate intestinal bleeding

**RIBBONS:** Stringy or ribbon-like. Gut inflammation; constipation from lack of water, low fiber or FODMAP intolerance, low stomach acid or enzymes; dysbiosis; possibly intestinal parasites (if cramping, nausea are at play).

**PEBBLES:** Constipation, lack of fiber, low levels healthy bacteria, antibiotics, low vagal nerve tone (brain gut), overtraining, under-sleeping, dehydration

**ROCK:** Constipation, low fiber intake, dehydration, dysbiosis, lack of sleep, mineral deficiency, stress, low stomach acid or low digestive enzymes, improper chewing, high protein without enough fiber or fat

**THE BIG DUMP:** Chronic constipation; megacolon; low stomach acid or enzymes; dysbiosis from stress, irregular eating habits, low vagal nerve tone

**MR. STANKY:** Something is toxic; Liver distress; Food intolerances

**MOLDING CLAY:** Gallbladder congestion; fat malabsorption

**PALE OR GRAY:** Bile deficiency; liver congestion or toxicity

**GREEN QUEASE:** Ate something green (can be normal); Maldigestion or malabsorption; Gallbladder congestion.

**YELLOW GREASE:** Low pancreatic enzymes & pancreatic dysfunction; Celiac disease; Blocked bile or pancreatic ducts (gallbladder or pancreas congestion); High fat diet

**SLIP & SLIDE:** Dysbiosis, bacterial gut infection, food intolerance or histamine intolerance, ate something funky, excessive stress, high fat diet & gallbladder malabsorption, SIBO

**LEFTOVERS:** Low digestive enzymes or low stomach acid, dysbiosis, food intolerances, high fiber diet

dr. lauryn
functional medicine. nutrition. therapy.
www.drlauryn.com
lauryn@drlauryn.com

What causes abnormal poop in the first place?

Stress. Generally, abnormal bowel habits are influenced by *stressors* like a lack of fiber, under-eating, dehydration, undersleeping, overtraining, eating too fast or on the go, *and* any "undigested" thoughts, beliefs, or emotions that you cannot absorb or eliminate. This is, at its most simple, a lack of balance.

## THE KEY TO A HAPPY GUT: HOMEOSTASIS

Like all things in the natural world, your body (and your gut microbiome) desires homeostasis: Balance, a lack of disease, and a lack of too much unhealthy stress.

After skipping breakfast, your grumbling, imbalanced stomach lets you know it wants avocado toast, sunny side up, with egg on top.

When you're running on three hours of sleep after submitting your paper at 4 a.m., drooping eyelids and head nods demand shut-eye, no matter how much you fight it.

If you wear jeans on a 99-degree summer day, your body sends Mayday signals to your brain: "AC, ice water, and short-shorts—stat!" Broken bone? It screams, "Don't move me!"

Our bodies are extremely good at telling us what they want and when they want it to maintain homeostasis—as long as we listen.

If we *don't* listen to our body, or if our stress levels exceed our body's ability to adapt or recover to stress, then Isaac Newton's First Law of Motion goes into effect. Newton's First Law of Motion states: An object in motion stays in motion with the same speed and in the same direction unless acted upon by an unbalanced force." Put another way: a gut microbiome that is balanced stays balanced *unless* acted upon by unbalanced forces. Stress is one such imbalanced force.

## UNDERSTANDING STRESS

When you hear the word "stress," what comes to mind? Work or school deadlines? Financial strain? An argument with your significant other?

Contrary to popular belief, stress goes far beyond mental stress, such as the stress we feel when stuck in the five o'clock rush hour traffic or when our computer crashes.

Stress entails *both* mental and physical stresses that elevate our cortisol (stress hormones) and disrupt our natural homeostasis. For instance, a plant can be under stress in a drought. Your favorite Barbie doll encounters stress when your little brother rips her head off, and our body was under stress when we broke a bone, falling off the monkey bars in First Grade. Stress is everywhere. These things do not need a mindset or neural pathways to be under stress.

Likewise, you can be sitting on a beach in Tahiti, sipping a pina colada and reading a great book—seemingly without a care in the world—but your body can *still* be under physiological stress if you have an underlying parasite infection, you're sleep deprived, and running off three to four cups of coffee every day. The same goes for you at home, staring at screens for eight to ten hours for work, or if you have Vitamin B deficiency anemia and low melatonin production.

## STRESS DEFINED

Stress is defined as "any event, threat, or tension in which environmental demands, internal demands, or both, strain or exceed your body or your mind's ability to adapt or recover from that stress."

Repeat: stress is defined as "any event, threat, or tension in which environmental demands, internal demands, or both, strain or exceed your body or your mind's ability to adapt or recover from that stress."

Stress most often arises in your life when something that you, or your body, cares about is at stake.

For example, if your computer crashes and you lose your thirty-page report due in 12 hours, stress arises. Why? You *care* about making a good grade. Stress arises in your body if you haven't eaten in 72 hours. This stress comes because your body *cares* about having enough energy to keep your cellular processes working in tip-top shape. And stress arises in your gut if you catch a cold and take antibiotics as a first line of defense. Your gut cares about having a thriving army of gut microbes to defend against pathogens. Antibiotics knock out both the good guys and bad guys.

Stress in our bodies and gut biomes is sort of like what happens if you poke a sleeping wasp nest. Prior to poking the nest, you would never know wasps lived inside. No signs of intelligent life anywhere. But say you take a stick from the yard, then jab that nest; what happens? You suddenly find yourself under siege from angry wasps attacking from every direction!

Stress is a normal part of life, and we can handle and adapt to a tremendous amount of stress without necessarily feeling negative side effects—like those all-nighter study sessions in grad school, reading a depressing news headline (or five of them) every day on our newsfeed, drinking three cups of coffee daily, or coming into contact with an ill person, but not getting sick if we wash our hands well and get a little extra sleep. However, just like that wasp nest, if we give our bodies one too many jabs, we disturb our microbial balance inside, sending inflammatory signals from the brain to the gut, and vice versa, from the gut to the brain.

## MODERN STRESS STINKS (FOR OUR GUT HEALTH).

Unfortunately, the Westernized world in which we live today stands in complete opposition to how our human genes (and guts) are innately wired to survive and thrive.

Let me ask you a question, why is it that our great-grandparents:

- Ate foods like steak and potatoes;
- Smoked cigarettes;
- Worked hard for very little pay;
- *NEVER* went to the gym a day in their life?

And yet, they were three times less likely to be overweight or experience the diseases many face today, like cancer, heart disease, and diabetes.

Meanwhile, in our generation, we live during the worst health epidemic of all human time—more than one in two Americans faces gut-related chronic diseases and health conditions, unlike any experienced human history. Today, the number one cause of death is not "old age," tuberculosis, infant mortality, or getting eaten by a sabertooth tiger like our ancestors. Instead, preventable lifestyle-induced diseases such as heart disease, stroke, cancer, Alzheimer's, and diabetes lead the way. In fact, the amount of money that goes towards treating metabolic diseases in the US every year is enough to cure world hunger, revealing our country as the "least healthy" of all developed nations.

By age 44, the average American will have six diagnoses to their name, from migraines to allergies, autoimmune disease, and cancer. Gen Z (kids born between 1996-2010) is the first generation not expected to outlive their parents—or at least live a quality life into old age (unless relying on insulin pumps, CPAP machines, and anxiety pills is how you define quality).

Is this because we are lazy, lack health information, and all eat McDonald's and Hershey's candy bars? Possibly, but not necessarily. We currently have 24/7 access to Dr. Google, gyms on every corner, and gluten-free everything. One in three people is on a diet at any given time in the U.S., with low-carb lifestyles leading the way, and more than 80 percent of Americans report that they seek to limit sugar and make "good choices" on a daily basis (10). So why is this not adding up to our health as a whole? Three words: *bad gut health*. A disrupted second brain.

Physically, our gut microbiomes have significantly changed over the past 100 years—something research has coined the "disappearing gut microbiome theory." It's been estimated that humans today have 40 percent less healthy, diverse gut bacteria than our ancestors, and if there is one thing you'll learn from this book as we go along, it is this: Health is an inside job. This entails proper digestion, absorption, a strong (gut) immune system, and microbial diversity and balance.

## BIG CHANGES TO THE HUMAN GUT TODAY

Research shows that when people move to the US, they almost immediately begin losing their native microbes and start inheriting a new microbiome correlated with obesity, autoimmunity, neuro-degeneration, and illness susceptibility—and their guts contain less diverse and fewer strains of bacteria

During the previous two hundred thousand years of life on earth, humans worked and played during the daylight hours, and rested and de-stressed at night. Humans also lived in strong tribes and bonded communities, ate natural (unprocessed) seasonal and regional foods, and found meaning and purpose in spirituality, nature, work, and family.

It wasn't until the last two hundred years—a couple of inches on the hundred-yard football field timeline of humanity—that the chronic disease epidemic came onto the scene. Although the human genome has not significantly changed, our lifestyles and gut microbiota have. Our 21st Century lifestyles are the nemesis of a healthy, balanced biome. Some examples and manifestations of this include:

- Being trapped indoors for 22-23 hours per day;
- Consume convenience frankenfoods in packages and drive-thrus;
- We sit for 12-plus hours per day;
- Often we eat the same things with little rotation or seasonal variety;
- We are always on the go—eating on the go, texting on the go;
- We look at artificial blue light an average of 6-11 hours every day—tricking our brains into thinking it's daytime around the clock.

So, on that note, let's take a little look at some of our gut health essentials and how these run in juxtaposition to our regular habits, especially when compared to our primitive ancestors and the environments in which our guts evolved:

- Our guts evolved to process nutrient-dense, real foods (grass-fed wild animals, poultry, and seafood; fermented foods, organic fruits, and veggies; healthy traditional fats; grass-fed full-fat raw dairy);
- High fiber intake (prebiotics);
- Clean water;
- Natural sunlight and clean air;
- Quality sleep and rest, in sync with the day/night cycle;
- Variety of movement (walking, sprinting, lifting heavy things) and play;
- Safe, healthy environment;
- Community and tribe;
- Purpose/meaning and work;
- Mental and emotional stability;

Our ancestors were not stress-free. However, unlike we modern-day humans who face these daily environmental and physiological health stressors, like pesticides and heavy metals in food and water, air pollution, EMF waves, and blue light exposure, the primary stressors of the long-ago past entailed the occasional natural disasters (for example, storms and earthquakes), wild predators, food scarcity (caused by drought and seasonal changes,) and relationship or tribal disputes. Our bodies are under daily siege, often from factors we can't even see or understand.

The Hadza tribe, modern-day hunter-gatherers living in Tanzania, are a perfect example of the health of a pre-modern way of life. Studies comparing the gut microbiomes of the Hazda people to the average Westerner found that the gut microbiomes of this tribe are far more diverse and even contain strains of bacteria associated with disease in the Western world. However, despite their lack of access to medical care, they tend to live long, healthy, and productive lives thanks to their vast amount of gut bacteria and gut-friendly lifestyles, which include maintaining seasonal, rotating diets, high prebiotic fiber intake (approximately 100-150 grams daily), circadian rhythm homeostasis (governed by a healthy sleep cycle), and strong tribal, community bonds.

Other studies comparing the gut bacteria profiles of those in urbanized cities to those in rural towns also find a distinct difference. We don't have to live on a remote island to experience this shift.For example, children living in a city versus a rural town often experience a significant decrease in short-chain fatty acids (essential for degrading unhealthy gut bacteria) and bacterial diversity. City dwellers, in general, also have a significant decrease in short-chain fatty acids and bacteria that digest fiber and plants and keep inflammation at bay, essential for feeding probiotic-rich bacteria. Our imbalanced, hectic lifestyles and diets are the scourge of a healthy, balanced biome.

The famous Pottenger's Cats experiment (1932-1942) illustrates how health degeneration can happen simply as a by-product of modern-day living and a lifestyle and environment not conducive to our innate human wiring. In the experiment, physician Dr. Francis Pottenger studied how diet and lifestyle affected four generations of cats. He divided the cats into two separate groups:

> **Cat Group #1:** Ate a processed food, pseudo-healthy diet—the equivalent to eating dry salads with chicken breast every day for lunch, artificially sweetened protein powders, and the whole grain cereals and boxed organic crackers sold at Whole Foods Market (read: not nutrient-dense);
>
> **Cat Group #2:** Ate an ancestral diet with nutrient-dense foods that cats had thrived upon for years (including raw milk, raw meats, and cod liver oil).

**The Findings:** the cats fed the all-raw diet were healthy, while the cats fed the cooked meat diet developed a slew of health problems. By the end of the first generation, the cats started to develop degenerative diseases and became quite lazy. By the end of the second generation, the cats had developed degenerative diseases by mid-life and started losing their coordination. By the end of the third generation, the cats had developed all sorts of issues, including blindness and weakness, shorter life spans, infertility, gut issues, skin diseases, allergies, arthritis, osteoporosis, and the inability to jump.

**Conclusion:** Modern living, with its many stressors, is not conducive to being a cat, let alone a human being, with many, many more stressors than your average cat.

Have you ever wondered how "bad health" actually happens as a result of stress? How does looking at blue light screens, reading a news headline about the latest political debate on Capitol Hill, eating an entire three-course meal in your car on the go, or drinking an extra shot of espresso with Half-and-Half creamer cause disease or inflammation? I mean, isn't stress inevitable?

*Enter: The Gut-Brain connection. Your Second Brain.*

# GUT CHECK POINT:

Stress—both mental and physical—is the number one driver of gut problems, including gut-immune, gut-hormone, gut-skin, gut-brain, and other gut-related conditions.

## REFERENCES


1. Kato-Kataoka, A., Nishida, K., Takada, M., Kawai, M., Kikuchi-Hayakawa, H., Suda, K., Rokutan, K. (2016). Fermented Milk Containing Lactobacillus casei Strain Shirota Preserves the Diversity of the Gut Microbiota and Relieves Abdominal Dysfunction in Healthy Medical Students Exposed to Academic Stress. *Applied and environmental microbiology, 82*(12), 3649–3658. doi:10.1128/AEM.04134-15
2. Martin, C. R., Osadchiy, V., Kalani, A., & Mayer, E. A. (2018). The Brain-Gut-Microbiome Axis. *Cellular and molecular gastroenterology and hepatology, 6*(2), 133–148. doi:10.1016/j.jcmgh.2018.04.003

3. Banerjee, A., Sarkhel, S., Sarkar, R., & Dhali, G. K. (2017). Anxiety and Depression in Irritable Bowel Syndrome. *Indian journal of psychological medicine, 39*(6), 741–745. doi:10.4103/IJPSYM.IJPSYM_46_17

4. Lau, N. M., Green, P. H., Taylor, A. K., Hellberg, D., Ajamian, M., Tan, C. Z., ... Alaedini, A. (2013). Markers of Celiac Disease and Gluten Sensitivity in Children with Autism. *PloS one, 8*(6), e66155. doi:10.1371/journal.pone.0066155

5. Smits, Samuel & Leach, Jeff & Sonnenburg, Erica & Gonzalez, Carlos & Lichtman, Joshua & Reid, Gregor & Knight, Rob & Manjurano, Alphaxard & Changalucha, John & Elias, Joshua & Dominguez-Bello, Maria & Sonnenburg, Justin. (2017). Seasonal cycling in the gut microbiome of the Hadza hunter-gatherers of Tanzania. Science. 357. 802-806. 10.1126/science.aan4834.

6. Ayeni, Funmilola & Biagi, Elena & Rampelli, Simone & Fiori, Jessica & Soverini, Matteo & Audu, Haruna & Cristino, Sandra & Caporali, Leonardo & Schnorr, Stephanie & Carelli, Valerio & Brigidi, Patrizia & Candela, Marco & Turroni, Silvia. (2018). Infant and Adult Gut Microbiome and Metabolome in Rural Bassa and Urban Settlers from Nigeria. Cell reports. 23. 3056-3067. 10.1016/j.celrep.2018.05.018.

7. De Filippo, C., Di Paola, M., Ramazzotti, M., Albanese, D., Pieraccini, G., Banci, E., ... Lionetti, P. (2017). Diet, Environments, and Gut Microbiota. A Preliminary Investigation in Children Living in Rural and Urban Burkina Faso and Italy. *Frontiers in microbiology, 8,* 1979. doi:10.3389/fmicb.2017.01979

8. Pottenger, F. 1983. Pottenger's Cats: A Study in Nutrition. Price-Pottenger Nutrition Foundation, Inc.

9. Healthline. 2020. American Gut Check. https://www.healthline.com/health/american-gut-check#9

10. International Food Information Council. 2018. 2018 Food & Health Survey. https://foodinsight.org/thanks-for-your-interest-in-the-2018-food-health-survey/

11. Vangay P, Johnson AJ, Ward TL, *et al.* US Immigration Westernizes the Human Gut Microbiome. *Cell.* 2018;175(4):962-972.e10. doi:10.1016/j.cell.2018.10.029

12. A. van der Kolk, B. 2014. The Body Keeps the Score. Penguin Random House Company.

13. Stevens, J. S., Jovanovic, T., Fani, N., Ely, T. D., Glover, E. M., Bradley, B., & Ressler, K. J. (2013). Disrupted amygdala-prefrontal functional connectivity in civilian women with posttraumatic stress disorder. *Journal of psychiatric research, 47*(10), 1469–1478. https://doi.org/10.1016/j.jpsychires.2013.05.031

14. Díaz-Garrido N, Badia J, Baldomà L. Microbiota-derived extracellular vesicles in interkingdom communication in the gut. J Extracell Vesicles. 2021 Nov;10(13):e12161. doi: 10.1002/jev2.12161. PMID: 34738337; PMCID: PMC8568775.

# PART TWO: PRINCIPLES, ASSESSMENTS, AND EXPERIMENTS

# CHAPTER 5:
# PSST! YOUR SECOND BRAIN IS SPEAKING. ARE YOU LISTENING?

*Backstage. Sixth Grade talent show. A star is about to be born.*

Heart pumping. Stomach fluttering. Thoughts running—rehearsing my choreography and Shania Twain's *Man I Feel Like a Woman* lyrics in my head as Blake Mason wowed and dazzled the audience with his Houdini-worthy magic tricks.

"Psst! You're up, kid! Two minutes!" Whispers Mr. Thomas, the nerdy backstage manager, looking up from his clipboard, glasses dropping to his nose.

By now, by heart is THUMPING, palms sweating, breath shortening, and butterflies—more like wasps— swarming. Then, my stomach starts churning.

"I uhh... I uhh... gotta go!" I said, beelining it to the loo.

Sixty seconds later, relieved, I'm ready to go.

Back to my spot. Center stage. X marks the spot.

Lights. Camera. Action.

# YOUR GUT IS A SMART COOKIE

Your gut is your Second Brain.

Ever experienced butterflies in your stomach? Boom! Gut-brain connection! Just like how you have probably only been able to think about how much your tummy hurts after you get food poisoning or how hungry you are if you haven't eaten in a while.

The gut-brain axis explains why, when study subjects drank a 300-calorie milkshake, but one half of the group believed the shake was a 140-calorie "Sensishake," while the other half believed the shake was a delicious 600-calorie "Indulgent Shake"—each group experienced a completely different metabolic response. The dieters experienced three times more hunger, and their metabolism went into "dieting mode," whereas the "Indulgent Shakers" walked away more nourished and satisfied.

The gut-brain axis also explains why kids with peanut allergies have been shown to overcome them when they think positive thoughts. In one experiment on overcoming peanut allergies, researchers gave 25 kids permission to feel good during the challenge—telling them that the re-introduction would be a positive experience. They told the other 25 kids that the food reintroduction would be challenging and they would probably experience food allergy symptoms. The result? Those challenged by the researchers to believe the experiment would be positive experienced less stress and food allergy flares.

Belief changes physiology. Whatever is going on inside your gut affects your brain, just like whatever is going on inside your brain—from perceived stress to feelings of peacefulness and homeostasis—affects your gut and total body health.

Enter: "German New Medicine" (GNM), also known as "The New Medicine," "German Healing Knowledge" (GHK), or as I call it, the "Gut-Brain Connection." The Gut-Brain Connection is an entirely different paradigm of all diseases and symptoms in the physical body as well as mental health and behavioral issues.

# THE GUT-BRAIN CONNECTION

I want to start this explanation of The Gut-Brain Connection with a disclaimer: What I am about to share with you is as mind-blowing and perhaps as controversial as when humans first learned that the world was round—not flat. However, I share it with you because it has been one of the most transformational tools for gut optimization for my patients in my clinical practice.

Before we unpack it, I ask one thing of you: Have an open mind because if you do, your life will change in ways you never thought possible.

That said, I don't want you to believe simply anything. Skepticism is not only healthy but also necessary for intuitive discernment. I've been working with this information for several years and witnessed and studied hundreds of case examples. These experiences have left me with no choice but to believe it. Still, encourage you to find your own validity in your own life with your own symptoms.

Know that belief in this information is not necessary. Just like you don't have to believe in gravity or love, you can see and feel the effects. And yet, it's still a choice. If you want to believe in them, you have to realize that there are people who still think the world is flat, not round: This doesn't change the fact that the Earth is indeed round.

So, the "Gut-Brain Connection," what is it?

The "Gut Brain Connection" is a mind-body science for uncovering and addressing the "root causes" of chronic and acute illness, from broken bones and seasonal allergies to IBS, hypothyroidism, autoimmune disease, and cancer.

Inspired by a framework called German New Medicine that empowers clinicians and patients alike to understand and restore wellness via the Gut-Brain Connection, it is particularly effective for helping patients bust through any ceilings they've been hitting in their health.

# THE HISTORY OF THE "GUT BRAIN BREAKTHROUGH" (GERMAN NEW MEDICINE).

German New Medicine science was initially founded in the 1980s by Dr. Ryke Geerd Hamer, an allopathic medical doctor who began to incorporate the power of the brain in healing from physical illness, based on his own recovery experience from cancer.

Dr. Hamer developed testicular cancer shortly after his son Dirk was killed in a tragic accident and died in his arms, which I do not need to explain was a significant emotional stressor in his life. It was during his treatment and recovery from cancer that Dr. Hamer began to question the "root causes" that preceded his disease. He soon realized that disease in the body is often preceded by *dis-ease*, or significant emotional stressor(s) and "conflict shock" in our lives via the Gut-Brain connection, not only for himself but his patients as well.

Being the data-driven doctor that he was, Dr. Hamer began studying his patients' CT brain scans, which eventually evolved into approximately sixty- to seventy thousand case studies on cancer and other diseases, demonstrating a completely different view on the creation of disease and illness.

Dr. Hamer discovered that patients with similar diseases had the same regions of their brain "highlighted" as concentric rings on the brain scans (known as "Hamer Focuses"), all depending on the shock and how the individual uniquely processed the shock.

For example, he found that testicular cancer patients, just like him, presented with concentric rings on the brain stem layer, and the shock manifested as a tumor in the testes. In contrast, patients with a cold or flu (a "stink" sensory conflict) had concentric rings on the prefrontal cortex brain region.

Instead of viewing disease as a biological malfunction, the Gut-Brain Connection framework views cancer, autoimmunity, diabetes, candida, and over a thousand other "diagnoses" as a byproduct of the body simply trying to heal after a significant stressor or "conflict shock" has occurred in your life.

These findings also inspired Dr. Hamer to establish five "Biological Laws," which I now call the Five Core Principles of the Gut-Brain Connection, explaining how it all works on a mental, emotional, and physiological level.

# CHAPTER 6:
# THE 5 CORE PRINCIPLES OF THE GUT-BRAIN CONNECTION

Are you ready to take back control? Through my work with clients and years of research and case study analysis, I have come to the realization of the Five Core Principles that define the Gut-Brain Connection and how these can be mastered, manipulated, and made to benefit us.

The first step to this is awareness. To master the Principles, you must first be aware of them and how they impact you, specifically. You must define your relationship with them, as this will go a long way toward your understanding and your ability to use them to take back control.

So, without further ado, let's dive straight into Principle 1.

# PRINCIPLE 1. "DIS-EASE" (STRESS) IN OUR LIVES SHOWS UP AS "DISEASE" (STRESS) IN THE BODY.

Every Significant Biological Special Program (SBS) or "disease"—from the common cold to cancer to food intolerances— originates from an SES (Significant Emotional Stressor) or unexpected "conflict shock" in the brain. To trigger the onset of a disease or health issue, the SES or shock is not just everyday stress—it's unexpected, dramatic, isolating, and/or you don't have any strategies to deal with the situation at hand.

Examples of common "conflict shocks" that may precede the onset of illness or a health issue include:

- Feeling stuck in your life—like a job you hate or a surprise pregnancy, when you really wanted to travel or start a business;
- A loss or separation. This could be a job or income loss, relationship, move, or loss of a loved one;
- Not feeling good enough or wanted, such as being "shocked" when the person you really like doesn't like you back, or your dad affirms that you'd be better off as an accountant than an actress, or your best friend stops talking to you;
- An "attack" such as an offending remark by a demanding boss, client, or partner;
- A long, drawn-out self-devaluation conflict (being hardest on yourself) and the "shock" of these feelings when you don't get into your dream school or don't get the job;
- Any life-threatening situation, for example, in an accident or during a medical emergency.

In turn, the brain downloads that "shock" or stressor and triggers the specific organs, tissues, or cells to react. The body becomes a *mirror* of what's really going on inside us.

Next, let's analyze what we call "conflict shocks." These conflict shocks are mental and spiritual conflicts or specific stressors that manifest in the body. The four primary types of conflict shock include:

## CONFLICT 1: *A "MORSEL CONFLICT"*

A morsel is a survival lifeline or sustenance, such as food, relationships, jobs and finances, family connection, and health in the body. Digestion problems, eating disorders, and throat and thyroid disorders are often "morsel conflicts."

**Morsel Conflict Examples:**

- **Not being able to digest a morsel:** This can include taking on too much to handle, losing a job, parents' divorce, or hearing the news that your best friend is sleeping with your partner. The morsel (conflict) gets stuck in your body. Bloating is common here.
- **Inability to catch a morsel** for "survival." This may include relationships that "never work out for you," an inability to make enough money, and your body not healing or losing weight no matter how hard you try. In these situations, it is as if you are striving to catch a rabbit you can't get your hands on. In such situations, asthma and lung-related issues often arise.
- **Inability to get rid of or eliminate a morsel,** like a toxic relationship, a nagging parent, or feeling stuck in a season of life. Voila: constipation.
- **Inability to swallow a morsel,** such as a mean comment made about you on social media, learning your parents are getting a divorce after twenty years of marriage, relocating cities for your spouse's job (when you weren't ready to move), or never feeling like your voice is heard. Hello, thyroid issues!

## CONFLICT 2: *ATTACK OR FEAR OF BEING ATTACKED CONFLICT*

This conflict is exactly what it sounds like: Feeling like others, or the world, is working against you. The Attack Conflict is also related to the physical integrity of the organism and often involves organs involved with "protecting ourselves." Skin symptoms are huge here—especially acne, eczema, rashes, skin cancer, and chronic dry and flaky skin. No wonder, then, so many teenagers develop acne! Teenagers exist in that awkward stage of life where they are in the process of developing their identity and may fear being rejected or judged by their appearance. As a result, it affects their skin, which is the first barrier and protection that the body has. Have you ever wondered why you magically seem to develop spots when you are stressed or anxious?

Other organs involved are the peritoneum (the sack around the guts), often resulting in a leaky gut; pleura—the sack around the lungs, related to bronchitis, coughing, or pneumonia; the pericardium—the sack around the heart that may result in shortness of breath, swelling or heart palpitations under stress; the amniotic sac around the uterus, linked to infertility under conflict, and the meninges around the brain related to fatigue, headaches, or difficulty concentrating.

**Attack Conflict Examples:**

- **Knife in the back:** A friend that backstabs you or gossips about you, a colleague or employee that steals from you or does not keep their word.
- **Being rejected or the fear of rejection:** "I would go back to middle school," said no one, ever.
- **Verbal abuse** or being cut down by others, such as a parent, teacher, coach, or peers.
- **Fear of Being Injured, Polluted, or Soiled:** Figuratively, this may look like fear of losing your job or your status on social media, feeling threatened, or fear of losing everything you've worked for when an ACL tear takes you out of your soccer season.
- **Nest Conflict:** Fear of being "attacked" or seen as not being a good parent by other parents. Or, it could be a fear of loneliness after your youngest child flies away from the "nest," leaving you behind, or after the loss of your dog. It could also be the perceived attack of your "nest" by infertility and an inability to conceive. Finally, it could be a loss from the nest through an unexpected death, divorce, or even a job transfer.

## CONFLICT 3: SELF-DEVALUATION/SELF-ESTEEM CONFLICT

The Self-Devaluation conflict is experienced as a byproduct of humiliation, abuse, failure, poor performance, or feelings of shame, guilt, or "not being good enough." Self-Devaluation conflicts are notorious for driving autoimmune disease (the degradation of self), osteoporosis and bone, tissue, and joint issues—from broken bones to arthritis, strains, sprains, chronic back pain, cysts, knee problems, or even pelvic bone area issues, which is the house of the reproductive organs and sexual Self-Devaluation and insecurity.

**Examples of Self-Devaluation Conflict:**

- **"Not good enough":** Are you constantly comparing yourself to others? Growing up, did you live in the shadow of your older sibling or never measure up to your dad's or mom's standards? This could explain a later diagnosis of celiac disease, Hashimoto's, or Lupus.
- **Feeling left out:** We all experience this at one time or another; however, if it's been thematic in your life or around a particularly sensitive topic for you. This feeling may arise from "all your friends" getting married or having babies except for you, or you were the "odd kid out" in middle school, which has plagued you for the rest of your life. This feeling can be more of a Self-Devaluation and disease-driving conflict.
- **Poor boundaries:** Have you ever wondered why women are more often prone to autoimmune diseases than men? Stereotypically, women are also more prone to be people pleasers or allow others to "walk over us."

## CONFLICT 4: *TERRITORY AND SEPARATION*

Territorial and separation conflicts involve the sensory perception of the environment, communication, social behavior, and interactions. They are related to defining territories and learning how to interact as well as with separation issues. The cortex is the part of the brain concerned with the social environment or your ability to deal with other people and "the outside world." The key symptoms involved include brain function (i.e., brain fog, focus, headaches), while the key organs impacted include the ducts of your body, like your breast glands and ducts, your gallbladder and liver ducts, pancreatic ducts, etc. A territory and separation conflict, such as suddenly becoming an empty nester, a divorce, or a big move, can result in symptoms like diabetes and hypoglycemia, hair loss, brain fog, and poor detox ability. These issues are linked to fatigue, sluggish bowels, reduced neurological function, high levels of circulating histamine, and food intolerances. Tumor growth is also quite common with a territory or separation conflict, as discovered by Dr. Hamer upon the loss of his son.

**Examples of Territory and Separation Conflicts:**

- **Territorial threat, survival, anger, or rivalry:** This may include conflict with a boss, colleague, friend, or neighbor.
- **Loss or a change in your business,** such as a slower season at work, reduced or loss of income, getting fired, or walking away from your career to start something new.
- **Family division and separation:** This may include the division with a business partner, relationship, friend, family, divorce, or children leaving home.
- **Sexual frustration:** Feeling violated or a partner not meeting your needs.
- **Loneliness or lack of community and connectedness.**
- **Environmental threat:** Mold and toxins in the environment, growing up in a "rough" neighborhood, or a difficult neighbor in your apartment complex.
- **Motor issues:** A lack of mobility may result in you being trapped in a city or job you hate, unable to move or take a step forward, and disability or injury.

*The Bottom Line: The specific ways that conflict manifests in the body is 100 percent unique to you and the way your brain downloads or perceives a conflict when it occurs.*

It is also crucial to note that not all conflicts result in disease or health problems. Remember, to cause a lingering, unsolved health challenge, from hypothyroidism to acne to shortness of breath that won't go away; most diseases begin with a significant emotional stressor. An SES is an event, belief, or challenge that is *unexpected, dramatic, or isolating*, and you have *no strategy* to deal with the situation. As a result, the SES remains not entirely processed. In the face of stress, be it mental or physical, our bodies and brains respond unconsciously, instinctively, automatically, and instantaneously. As a result, the brain sends signals via the Gut-Brain Connection down the vagus nerve to corresponding organs, tissues, and cells.

# PRINCIPLE 2.
# THE ONSET OF DISEASE AND SYMPTOMS HAPPENS IN TWO PHASES:

## *PHASE 1: **FIGHT OR FLIGHT ("STRESS MODE")***

In the first phase, called "conflict active," the body enters permanent "stress mode," responding in much the same way as it would if it was fleeing a bear in the wild. In the fight or flight state, metabolism is rapidly and vastly increased, there is a sudden influx of energy, the need for food and sleep decreases (with regular waking up at around 3 a.m.), pulse rate increases, extremities become cold easily, and the body uses its reserves (energy and nutrients), especially if the stress period is prolonged.

When we enter "stress mode," specific areas of the brain are activated and begin sending inflammatory signals to specific tissues, organs, microbes, and cells. Specific areas are targeted depending on the specific type of stress. For example, "indigestible" conflict sends signals to the gut, later manifesting as IBS, bloating, SIBO, or constipation. CT brain scans show concentric rings in certain areas of the brain correlated with specific body organs and tissues where inflammation or disease may manifest.

## *PHASE 2: **SYMPTOMS ARISE***

In the second phase, "conflict resolution," the initial triggering stressor calms down, and you go into "parasympathetic" (less stressed) mode. The body begins to take in everything that just happened, and you finally *feel* the ankle you just sprained or the injuries you suffered.

Interestingly, the development of the symptoms always matches the development of the conflict and the type of conflict. For example, sudden conflict means sudden illness, and building/long-term conflict means disease builds over time.

This is where symptoms of all sorts unfold, and you typically get diagnosed with *something*, be it tumors (cancer), cold and flu, chronic fatigue, acne, yeast infections, anxiety, hair loss, thyroid flare, food intolerances, toxic mold illness, or lye disease. During this phase, you need to regain energy, and you also need correct mental, emotional, and nutritional support.

During Phase 2, you have two options after symptoms arise: *Recover or continue being sick*. Chronic illness is often a byproduct of unresolved (tissue, organ, bacterial, and cellular level) stress because otherwise, the body already has the perfect blueprint of health and healing. For example, break a bone and slap a cast on it, and in six to eight weeks, your bone is "healed." Your body naturally wants to heal and resolve the issues in your tissues unless the stressors go unaddressed.

## PRINCIPLE 3. THE MIND, BODY, AND SPIRIT ARE CONNECTED.

Physical disease is derived from "dis-ease" in the mind and spirit. Likewise, physical dis-ease (such as sleep deprivation or lack of exercise) also disrupts peace and causes distress in the mind and spirit.

Here, it is crucial to recognize the innate and real connections between the working of your brain, your mental state, and the way your body operates. The tangible connection between your brain as the CPU of your body and the gut as the fuel intake system means that an imbalance in one naturally affects the other. Don't ignore symptoms; look for trends and patterns that emerge between how you feel psychologically and your health physiologically. If you keep a log, these trends will become glaringly obvious.

There's a reason the gut is called the Second Brain. This term is growing in popularity because we are finally starting to develop an understanding of the impact our gut can have on the way we think. We are barely scratching the surface, and if you think about the surge in the understanding of neuroscience in recent years, gut science, as it pertains to emotional states, is fast growing in influence and understanding along much the same lines.

# PRINCIPLE 4. GUT BACTERIA (MICROBES) DRIVE DISEASE & HEALING.

Gut bacteria are *not* active when the body is healthy. They are balanced and at peace. However, after fight or flight mode, gut microbes go to work to heal, which is why gut issues and stress go hand in hand. Microbes don't cause diseases–instead, they play a crucial role during the healing phase. After the moment any stress or conflict is "resolved" (fight or flight is over), our fungi, bacteria, and viruses go to work. They become active and begin to assist the healing process. Gut "problems," like SIBO, candida, and dysbiosis, are often signs that the body is trying to heal and is failing to do so.

So, it is no wonder that when we go to the hospital or to the doctor with any illness, we are asked questions about our diet and often given advice as to what we should eat. Our guts are immensely powerful tools for healing. It is the center through which all nutrition enters our bodies, and the conditions and state of our microbiome play an intuitive role in how the nutrients we need to heal our bodies are absorbed into the bloodstream. So, help it by creating the right conditions for your microbiome and your gut to thrive.

To do this, it pays to understand more about your microbiome. Everyone is different. No two people digest food in the same way. Some are better at metabolizing sugars, others fat or lipids. It helps significantly if you understand what the colony of bacteria living in your gut likes to eat so that you can feed it best and allow your body to thrive.

To help, there are all sorts of tests you can take that will analyze your microbiome and give you advice on what you should eat more of and what you should look to have less of.

## PRINCIPLE 5. DISEASE AND SYMPTOMS ARE A WAY YOUR BODY IS SPEAKING TO YOU.

"Knock knock. Please listen. I want to help you." Our bodies want to work *for us, not against us*. Our bodies are resilient, hardy, and geared towards survival as a result of millions of years of evolution.

They are constantly speaking: *My back muscles are tight from overuse; I feel lightheaded and hangry; I have pent-up energy from sitting all day; I don't feel good when you eat an entire pint of ice cream; I feel brain foggy in this moldy space.*

Sometimes, though, and likely more often than we like to admit, we just aren't listening–and we really should! Any disease or symptoms we experience are opportunities to get curious about what our body is trying to tell us, i.e., what emotional triggers or stressful events have happened lately? Once resolved, the body is better able to heal.

Cravings, intrusive thoughts, urges... none of these things are accidents. Our brains are intense chemical factories, and every thought is governed by a series of chemical releases and electrical impulses, and *something sparks that impulse*. It rarely happens by accident. This is your body's way of talking to you, so take note. You don't need to act on every impulse, but it pays to get curious and ask: *Why* am I having this thought? What is my body trying to tell me? How can I help my body as it tries to heal me? What does it need? Once you crack this code, you are well on the way to a happier, healthier you.

# CHAPTER 7:
# THE FIVE PRINCIPLES IN ACTION

There you have it. The Five Core Principles of the Gut-Brain Connection.

Don't just take my word for it. Case studies—others' stories—are often the best way to see these 5 Biological Laws at play.

## "I'M FAT"

During Fourth Grade recess when the Queen Bee told me I was fat and should lose weight, this was SHOCKING and STRESSFUL.

I instantly felt a lack of self-worth; I was sad, hurt, and overwhelmed, and I could not fully digest, swallow, or process the information. As a result, this unprocessed mini-trauma or stressful event went "silent" for years, the words *you're not good enough* subconsciously etched in my brain.

Instead of working through the stressor and speaking up to the Queen Bee, the stressor took root in my body and soon manifested as an **eating disorder and IBS**, representing a self-worth and indigestible conflict that would remain stuck in my body for years.

Here, Principles 1 and 3 came into play, where a conflict created a situation that my body manifested into disease and, in turn, had devastating consequences on my mind, body, and spirit, creating a spiral of deteriorating health that took years, and a vast amount of therapy and treatment, to solve.

# BACON INTOLERANCE BECKY

Becky developed, seemingly out of nowhere, a sudden bacon intolerance. Thing is, she loved bacon and had been eating it regularly for years. What was once her go-to comfort food had not become her discomfort food, causing her stomach pain and a variety of other symptoms, not least of which impacted her mental state. So, what was going on?

Well, given that something drastic had changed, and this was seemingly not an allergy or intolerance as it would likely have emerged years earlier, and with other, similar foods, we realized that there must have been a stressor.

Remember, your get is your Second Brain, and making it only natural that an event that leaves a bad taste in your mouth can also have a remarkable, subconscious impact on your eating habits.

When she did reflective work to figure out what stressors were going on in her life preceding her bacon intolerance, she realized that the moment that her marriage broke down and she discovered that her husband had been cheating on her was a time that she was cooking bacon. Due to the inextricable link between the two, her mind and her gut had associated this traumatic life event, or stressor, with the taste and smell of bacon, causing an involuntary reaction to a food that once brought her joy. I'm sure we have all had those moments where we say, "No, I can't eat that, it reminds me of..."

Game set match! Her body locked her issues into her tissues. Principle 2 in action

# JENNIE'S RANDOM UTI

"Dr. Lauryn, I haven't had a UTI in years! What should I do?" a patient, Jennie, messaged me one day.

Of course, my "go-to's" as a clinician are the Urinary Tract Infection staple remedies: cranberry, D-Mannose, Uva Ursi, and probiotics.

However, when we "did the work" and brainstormed what, if any, stressors were present prior to her getting a UTI, we realized that for the entire past week, she had been experiencing intense conflict with her husband–her sexual partner. Well, lo and behold! UTIs are related to "territorial" or "separation" conflicts, particularly with our significant others.

The Gut-Brain Connection, and Principle 2, strike again.

## DAN'S SKIN RASH

Skin "problems" are often linked to an attack conflict—something Dan knew all too well. Eight years earlier, he'd been involved in a nasty lawsuit with the partner in his business that resulted in significant financial loss and a valued friendship loss in one go.

Ironically, around the same time—eight years ago—he also recalled developing a random skin rash that continued to flare every so often to this day, with no apparent rhyme or reason.

Was it gluten? Dairy? Alcohol? Sugar? Mold? He couldn't put his finger on it.

Remember Principle 1 and Attack Conflict. Every time his brain was reminded of the same emotions he'd experienced during the skin rash onset eight years previously, his skin would flare again. Anger and hurt were not his best friends—especially if he felt like someone was having a "go" at him, like when his wife made a negative comment about him not taking out the trash, or a tough day at work with a negative client on the other end of the phone.

Here, Principles 1 and 3 work in harmony to create disharmony; an Attack Conflict anchor and amplified by the mind, body, and spiritual Gut-Brain Connection created the perfect storm, creating the eight-year-long skin rash echo.

## KAITLYN'S HAIR LOSS

Kaitlyn's hair was falling out in clumps. At age 33 and with no known thyroid disorder, there was no explanation for it–except for that move to the opposite end of the country–from Washington to Florida–leaving her friends, church, and community of 13 years behind. Oh, and that breakup with her fiancé and boyfriend of five years. He was not the one, and she knew it, but that didn't make it any easier.

These separation conflicts resulted in her body's subconscious separation from her hair and Principles 1, 2, and 3, all working in concert to manifest an extreme, physical reaction.

## PHOEBE'S SIBO AND BLOATING

Phoebe was bloated. All the time. On the surface, she was, to all intents and purposes, doing "all the things," including a low FODMAP diet, supplementing to boost her enzymes, SIBO and candida, therapy and treatment, and the list goes on...

However, a key part of my treatment is understanding the stressors and unique individual circumstances in one's life, and in Phoebe's, she was as bloated in her life as her stomach was. You see, in her life, she was well known for "all the things," only these things were for everyone else. She was living in cold, windy Chicago, attending college, and studying toward a major that she hated to please her dad—finance—while her heart's desire was to be a movie screenwriter in Los Angeles.

She was feeling, both mentally and physically, *very* bloated until, that is, she finally took the leap. Listened to her gut, and in turn, due to that Gut-Brain Connection, listened to her brain. Phoebe moved, quite suddenly, to L.A. to finish her last semester "abroad" and intern on the set of Hollywood studios.

The bloating that she experienced soon went away and never returned. By addressing her stressors and listening to her body, she managed an issue that had plagued her for years.

## SARAH'S INFERTILITY

Sarah had immense difficulty getting pregnant. She and her partner had tried everything—chaste tree berry, cutting the intense cardio, upping her calories, taking probiotics, eating organic foods, incorporating breathwork, and yoga. However, nothing was working.

Infertility is often related to a territorial conflict of some sort for either the woman, the man, or both. For instance, the "conflict" or fear of losing independence to some degree with the addition of a new baby to the mix. Or, it could be a territorial conflict involving a relationship conflict of some sort.

So, when I told her this, Sarah opened up, and she revealed to me that her husband was not completely on board. He felt increased pressure to provide and work harder at the mere thought of multiplying their family and was unsure if he could do it.

Ultimately, on as much my advice as her own initiative, Sarah had a conversation with him. The couple came together to make a game plan to feel more prepared on the financial front.

Within two weeks, she was pregnant.

## SUMMARY: GREEN JUICE, KETO, AND PROBIOTICS WILL ONLY GET YOU SO FAR.

The stories could go on. The truth is, we are just getting started. I have included an entire list of common conditions and the associated conflicts in the Resources section at the end of this book for your reference. For example, thyroid-related problems are often due to a "morsel conflict"—the inability-to-get-a-chunk-in-or-out conflict. Sinus congestion is related to a "stink conflict," where something stinks or is lousy in your life, such as when the stock market drops, you don't get picked for something you want, or you receive a rude or terse email. If the brain interprets this conflict as a "shock," once the conflict seemingly gets resolved is the moment you catch a cold.

Unfortunately, most conventional medicine modalities and even functional medicine focus *primarily* on the physical aspects of healing—prescriptions, lab tests, diets, supplements, exercise, sleep, and protocols. This approach, however, almost completely neglects the fact that our unconscious mind runs 95 percent of our body, including our physical health, and has control over our thoughts, feelings, beliefs, emotions, sensory inputs, and perceived stress. Hence, green juice, anti-candida diets, and probiotics will only get you so far.

The cool thing? You hold within yourself a great power to heal your body with your mind. It all begins with *awareness*. Resolution from symptoms actually begins when we recognize the root causes behind our greatest health challenges. For example, say you experienced a significant attack conflict—a friend turns their back on you. This conflict catches you off guard. *You* maintain resentment, sadness, and hurt about the situation for years without realizing that it occurred at about the same time that your random adult acne began in your life. "Resolution" or "healing" may come from this disease when we "mend" the wound that was created at a brain level by forgiving the old friend or making ourselves move on.

Throughout the rest of this book, you will learn tools and strategies for not only identifying the root causes behind your greatest health challenges but optimizing the Gut-Brain Connection to be truly unstoppable.

You will achieve a Total Gut Reset.

## GUT CHECK POINT

Our brain and our gut run the body. Symptoms are a sign your body is trying to "heal" after a significant stressor or conflict shock and are often a metaphor for what is going on inside.

### REFERENCES


1. Laurent, H. K., Stroud, L. R., Brush, B., D'Angelo, C., & Granger, D. A. (2015). Secretory IgA reactivity to social threat in youth: Relations with HPA, ANS, and behavior. Psychoneuroendocrinology, 59, 81–90. https://doi.org/10.1016/j.psyneuen.2015.04.021
2. Crum AJ, Corbin WR, Brownell KD, Salovey P. Mind over milkshakes: mindsets, not just nutrients, determine ghrelin response. Health Psychol. 2011 Jul;30(4):424-9; discussion 430-1. doi: 10.1037/a0023467. PMID: 21574706.
3. Howe LC, Leibowitz KA, Perry MA, Bitler JM, Block W, Kaptchuk TJ, Nadeau KC, Crum AJ. Changing Patient Mindsets about Non-Life-Threatening Symptoms During Oral Immunotherapy: A Randomized Clinical Trial. J Allergy Clin Immunol Pract. 2019 May-Jun;7(5):1550-1559. doi: 10.1016/j.jaip.2019.01.022. Epub 2019 Jan 23. PMID: 30682576; PMCID: PMC6511320.

CHAPTER 8:

# HOW TO HEAL YOUR GUT: THE TOTAL GUT RESET.

Your genes are not your destiny. Your diagnosis is not your identity. A long-term disease or projected illness statistic does not have to be your outcome.

What if I told you that you hold within you the power to completely revolutionize your body and total health from the inside out?

You do.

## ALL. THE. THINGS. (DIDN'T CURE ME).

When I got really sick, I did everything my ten-plus years and thousands upon thousands of dollars of health and wellness education and academia had taught me to do:

- Low-glycemic carbs for hypoglycemia, then keto when that didn't work;
- Candida cleanses to kick my bloating, followed by a SIBO protocol to blast those little bacteria boogers in my small intestine;
- Boswellia AKBA and liposomal curcumin for inflammation;

- Antimicrobial herbs to kill bacteria—berberine, wormwood, grapefruit seed;
- Red light therapy for hypothyroidism;
- Homeopathics for migraines;
- Liver detox supplements and coffee enemas for mycotoxin illness and mold;
- Chlorella tablets, green juice, and infrared sauna for heavy metals;
- Ashwagandha and Rhodiola for my cortisol rollercoaster;
- Reiki, acupuncture, and limbic system training to calm the stress inside;
- Peppermint essential oil for asthma;
- Hyperbaric oxygen therapy and ozone treatment for the mini-stroke I got from contraindicating supplements;
- Glutathione IV therapy for autoimmune flares.

If a symptom flared, I found myself trying to suppress it as quickly as I could, turning to my inner circle of Facebook group forums, old textbooks and notes, PubMed, and, as a last resort, Dr. Google for the answers. Even though I was all about getting to the root cause, as my training had taught me, I also just wanted the fires inside me to stop.

*Please, God. Make it stop. Be Lord over my body.* I prayed often and fervently. At times, I felt as if my prayers bounced off the ceiling.

Certainly, some dietary interventions helped. Others made things worse. Some supplements worked, while others didn't. I met a lot of really nice holistic practitioners. But looking back on the experience (and my credit card bills), I can confidently say that more restrictions, more pills, and more appointments and therapies were not the answer.

In a year's time, seventy-five thousand dollars of hard-earned savings got me *through* the experience but didn't get me *over* it. In fact, nothing radical changed in my healing process until I said *enough* and decided to instead focus my energy on getting back to the basics.

## OVER IT!

*Kerplunk!* The trash sack hit the bottom of the dumpster, filled with the forty-plus different supplement bottles I'd ordered over the past 12 months, seeking the magic ingredient I seemingly could not find. I was so over it all. I hated taking 18 pills every day, not knowing which ones were working or not.

My fridge and pantry were also given a makeover. Tired of eating the same safe five foods every single day because they were all my body could tolerate, I hit the grocery store to find new foods to experiment with and expand my horizons. Even with my five safe foods that didn't spike histamine flares—rainbow chard, ground turkey, summer squash, coconut butter, and chicken—my body had not necessarily been getting better. I added foods like jicama, purple sweet potato, delicata squash, ground bison, halibut, coconut yogurt, and dark chocolate to my cart. What did I have to lose by trying new things?

The battle for my body had begun, and on the lifestyle front, I started sleeping more. I fought to get good rest to let my body heal, even when I'd wake up at 4 a.m. with my body in fight or flight mode. I stopped overtraining. I integrated yoga, fresh-air walks, and an actual training plan, giving up the chronic cardio and HIIT workouts.

For my mindset, I stopped researching. I broke up with Facebook and stopped turning to Dr. Google for every symptom. I also replaced my health-focused podcasts and Audible playlist, focusing on personal development, communication, prayer, spiritual growth, and mindlessly fun fiction.

Above all, I started believing that, when given the right tools, my body and my gut could and would heal. *Repeat: when given the right tools, the body innately wants to heal itself.*

Enter: the Total Gut Reset—the full-immersion journey I embarked upon to do just that when Dr. Google, kombucha, liver detox supplements, and doctors couldn't help.

The result? Within a matter of months, my body began to get back online. My shortness of breath became practically nonexistent. I didn't need coffee to provide me with energy. I no longer needed IBS bathroom trips (which had shot up to 14-plus times a day), and I went up by twenty much-needed pounds, slowing my catabolic muscle wasting and malabsorption, Just like others may naturally lose weight.

I had more light in my eyes, and I began to genuinely feel better.

The best part? The Total Gut Reset is not just my journey. It can be yours too.

## THE PROBLEM WITH MOST GUT HEALING PROTOCOLS–THE GUT-BRAIN FORMULA.

Many gut problems and related conditions fail to heal because the classic treatment model completely ignores the three steps for health optimization, the Gut-Brain Formula—the three essentials for transforming how you look, move, feel and think.

All too often, people end up with a medicine cabinet full of half-used supplements, overly restrictive no-FODMAP-no-oxalates-no-lectin-no-starch diets, and seven expensive lab tests, only to find themselves feeling exactly the same as when they started. They had failed to address the root cause mechanism(s) driving their symptoms.

This three-step Gut-Brain Formula is comprised of the following steps:

**Step 1: Tune into your gut;**

**Step 2: Take care of your gut;**

**Step 3: Trust your gut.**

How to do it? Just follow along; this book will take you on the journey to restore your Gut-Brain Connection.

## YOU CAN WRITE A NEW STORY FOR YOUR HEALTH

You have the ability to write a new story for your health, just as I did.

The moment I threw away all my supplements catapulted me into going beyond simply managing my symptoms or dealing with diagnoses. I *knew* shortness of breath, blood sugar imbalances, and loose, watery stools, and muscle wasting, bloating, constipation, and headaches were not my norm. Nor did they have to be for life. The same thing goes for you.

The remainder of this book is dedicated to helping you become the best version of yourself by guiding you in the play-by-play fundamentals and building up your toolbox to reset your gut health with the simple three-step process.

*Remember: Health is an inside job. To a Total Gut Reset, we go!*

## GUT CHECK POINT:

When given the right tools, the body innately wants to heal itself. Start with the three steps for a total gut reset, and you are well on your way.

# CHAPTER 9: TUNE INTO YOUR GUT

Welcome to your official Total Gut Reset and bus stop number one of the "Gut Brain Formula": Tune into your Gut. This first stop is all about tuning in to what your gut is trying to tell you with your baseline assessments.

The first steps are all about evaluation and assessment. Evaluation and assessments are essential for any goal-centered endeavor. In fitness, athletes test their mile time, max squat, bench press weight, or max heart rate during a HIIT workout. In relationships, couples assess their personal love language and communication style. In school, your math skills and skills at literary analysis were tested every few weeks to help ensure you were gaining the knowledge of calculus or the ability to read and think critically when reading Shakespeare. And if you have a sore throat, fever, and runny nose, a doctor may run a strep or flu test.

The principle is that if you don't know where you've come from, you don't know where you're going. The same principle applies to gut health—especially when we're talking about starting your Total Gut Reset journey.

Does the following sound familiar?

*Late-night Google search:* Natural candida remedies.

*Results:*

- Oregano oil,
- Coconut oil,
- Greek yogurt,
- Tea tree oil,
- Garlic,

- Apple cider vinegar,
- Probiotic suppositories and supplements,
- Boric acid,
- Vitamin C,
- Hydrogen peroxide.

Believe me, I have tried them all. Nothing worked–at least nothing worked a hundred percent.

The clincher? I didn't *just* have candida. I had mold and fungal overgrowth. I had small intestinal bacterial overgrowth (SIBO). I had a heavy metal overload. I had mass cell activation syndrome and Th1/Th2 immune dysregulation. I had Vitamin B2, manganese, Vitamin D, and Vitamin A deficiency. I had a leaky gut. I had unsolved "indigestible" or Mosel conflicts. My body stumped Dr. Google.

The truth is, I would never have discovered any of these facts until I actually learned how to tune in and stopped guessing and symptom chasing, trying to figure things out on my own—throwing money at random supplements on Amazon, hoping they would help, and restricting a new list of foods every week.

Tuning into your gut by testing, not guessing, is a fast-track way to stop shooting darts in the dark. Ideally, properly utilized testing methods can help you figure out your health conditions.

Although we cannot cover every single test and assessment out there, in this chapter, we will discuss a handful of essentials to save you both the time and money you might otherwise spend on tests that don't work. These essentials are:

- Assessment 1: The 5 Gut Types
- Assessment 2: Health Story Timeline
- Assessment 3: The Gut Check Method
- Assessment 4: The Golden Poo Challenge
- Assessment 5: Clinical Lab Tests

Next, we'll briefly discuss each of these assessments you can do at home, and how doing so will allow you to become your own personal health detective.

The cool thing? Most of these tests are completely free of charge, easy to complete, and arguably more accurate than even many fancy test kits and biohacking tools out there. For a complete overview and directions for each assessment, see the Resources section at the back of this book.

# ASSESSMENT 1: THE 5 GUT TYPES

You know your blood type. You might also know your body type and your skin type. But what about your Gut Type?

Knowing your Gut Type can help you and your practitioner identify the underlying cause(s) of ill health, as well as determine what further testing, nutrients, and supplements may be of benefit.

Most people have one of the following five main Gut Types, particularly when their body gets out of balance. The five Gut Types are:

1. Digestive Gut;
2. Immune Gut;
3. Detox Gut;
4. Hormonal and Metabolic Gut;
5. Inflamed Gut.

Each of the five Gut Types represents a variety of symptoms that stem from stress via the Gut-Brain Connection and manifest in that particular system.

A **Digestive Gut Type** presents with the most overt digestive problems, food problems, and gut-related symptoms, including constipation, bloating, irregular stools, nausea, IBS, IBD, SIBO, stomach pain, and fungal overgrowth (candida). However, as you have learned already, "gut issues" from stress go beyond bloating and constipation.

The **Immune Gut Type** tends to show up as skin problems, autoimmune conditions, allergies, asthma, sinus infections, or the common cold and flu.

A person with a **Detox Gut Type** has toxic overload and may present with a variety of seemingly unsolved symptoms that are not easily resolved by typical or holistic treatments. These symptoms may include fatigue unrelieved by sleep and coffee, brain fog, skin rashes and breakouts, IBS, and/or multiple sensitivities—to chemicals, foods, sounds, lights, people's energy, caffeine, alcohol, and/or smells. Detox Gut folks may have a history of mold exposure, Lyme disease, breast implant illness, or work in a "toxic" industry (like cosmetics or construction). They are also highly intuitive and sensitive themselves.

Hormonal and **Metabolic Gut Types** represent hormone and metabolic challenges, like infertility, PMS and estrogen dominance, low testosterone, thyroid disorders, diabetes, and pre-diabetes.

Finally, the **Inflamed Gut** is exactly what it sounds like—a cocktail of chronic inflammation and oxidative stress sprinkled with an extremely high helping of cortisol. Hello, chronic back pain, headaches, high blood pressure, heart disease, and neuroinflammation—ADD/ADHD, Alzheimer's, and anxiety.

Now, it is important to note that Your Gut Type is not fixed; it can change throughout your life, and varying Gut Type symptoms are simply just a metaphor—smoke signals—for stress that has previously occurred in the Gut-Brain Connection. "Stress" may be physical (such as eating cheeseburgers and Slushies every day for lunch), or "stress" may be mental and emotional.

Think about it: We all know a 90-year-old Uncle Joe who smokes cigars, eats bologna on white bread and orange soda, and sits in his "lazy boy" recliner every day of his life yet lives symptom-free, whereas 29-year-old Lauryn eats pristine, works out every day—sometimes twice-and takes boatloads of supplements, but gets diagnosed with over ten chronic diseases.

So, what is *really* happening here?

*Remember: Dis-ease in our lives can end up as disease in the body.*

## ISSUES IN OUR TISSUES

Interestingly, CT scans show that people with different Gut Types have inflammation in specific regions of their brain, correlated with their specific Gut Type at play. The brain is mapped for over a thousand different symptoms and conditions, from anxiety to insomnia, bloating, eating disorders, heart attacks, nasal congestion, and even cancer. Sort of like a tree that contains rings that tell its age, when a "conflict shock" or significant stressor occurs, your brain gets inflamed with concentric rings that then send a signal for specific symptoms to arise. Voila: Your Gut Type shines.

Even if you can't pinpoint or recall the specific stressor or trigger, often your symptoms will give you a clue about the specific conflict. While we don't have time to map out each of the thousand different symptoms and conditions, let's run through a prominent few.

## *DIGESTIVE GUT*

Bloating (associated with a Digestive Gut) often stems from an "indigestible" conflict" or "morsel conflict"—not being able to absorb or digest a morsel.

Examples of an "indigestible conflict" may be:

- Receiving a diagnosis, bad news, or something hard to "digest" or "swallow";
- Undigested anger or sadness, for instance, anger about a person (a family member, friend, neighbor, colleague, employee, supervisor, client, teacher, student, classmate, coach, doctor, authorities) or sadness about a situation;
- A parent for whom you can never measure up to their demands, no matter how hard you try.

Similarly, other gut issues like colitis, constipation, loose stools, and nausea, and eating issues, like food intolerances and disordered eating, stem from "indigestible conflicts."

Food intolerances with recurring diarrhea reveal that an "indigestible anger" related to a particular food (milk, nuts, wheat, seafood, a certain fruit or vegetable) has not been completely resolved—such as Bacon-Intolerant Becky.

## *IMMUNE GUT*

The Immune Gut is often related to an "attack conflict" or threat. Since the immune system is your body's number one "defense" system, acne may pop up if we feel bullied or poked fun of for what we look like–the curse of many a teenager.

Autoimmune disease is linked to a "self-degradation" (i.e., self-attack) conflict. The immune system degrades its own tissues just like we degrade ourselves with thoughts like "I'm not good enough," highlighted by inflammation in the frontal lobe—the brain region connected to negative self-talk.

Sinus and nasal congestion are related to a "stink conflict." The stink conflict translates into "smelling" trouble or a potential threat (an attack), for instance, "smelling" a competitor or an opponent at work, at school, at home, or in a relationship. Any offending situation that is perceived as "This stinks!" or "I am fed up with this!" also meets the stink conflict criteria—like cold winter days replacing warm summer sunshine, or being "left behind" by our mom for several days each week at a diaper-smelling daycare with 12 other strangers.

## DETOX GUT

The Detox Gut is all about the inability to eliminate properly (liver and gallbladder congestion) and also the "starvation" of several key nutrients, stopping us from functioning optimally.

Hence, symptoms that show up under the Detox Gut umbrella are closely related to "elimination" and "starvation" conflicts—figuratively, not being able to eliminate something in our lives (like a toxic relationship or job situation), or figuratively feeling like you are "starving," such as being put on a strict diet, broken family relationships growing up, feeling lonely, not being allowed to eat your favorite food, or unintentional weight loss. All of these have the potential to trigger the conflict. Since the liver and the gallbladder are the top detox organs, if you can't eliminate a situation or you suffer from "starvation," it may activate reduced gallbladder and liver function.

As for specific Detox Gut related conditions, like mold illness, mast cell activation syndrome, and Lyme disease (characterized by a wide array of signs and symptoms), each symptom is linked to a specific type of conflict that all stack on top of each other to generate a variety of illnesses and symptoms.

For example, when I was exposed to toxic mold, my body struggled with shortness of breath (a "death fright" conflict—around the same time that I started my first business and no longer had a steady paycheck), whereas another person exposed to toxic mold may experience significant IBS (an "indigestible conflict"), dizziness (from a "hearing conflict"; *something she can't believe she heard*), or skin rashes (an "attack" conflict).

*Again: Symptoms are often just representations and manifestations of the stressors going on in our lives and how our brain, at a psyche level, is processing it all.*

## HORMONAL AND METABOLIC GUT

Do water retention and swelling, bloating, weight gain, thyroid, and hormone imbalances sound familiar?

We often link these to a "slow metabolism," but according to the Gut-Brain Connection, these are actually related to a "kidney collecting tubule conflict," also known as a water retention conflict, where the kidney collecting tubules "tighten up" and where there is minimum fluid (urine) excretion and maximum fluid retention along with elevated kidney enzymes when in *deep* conflict—specifically an AIRE (Abandonment, Isolation, Refugee, Existence) conflict.

We need air(e) to survive. The kidney-collecting tubules are all about survival and our existence, and if we experience any one of these conflicts (Abandonment, Isolation, Refugee, Existence), water retention and swelling, bloating, and weight gain may easily show up.

With a kidney collecting tubule program, the biological meaning is understood within the context of evolution. When a fish has washed ashore, it is immediately tossed into a life-threatening predicament through water deprivation where its very existence is threatened; the fish is out of its element and elements. In order to prevent the organism from drying out, the cells of the kidney tubules quickly expand and swell with the biological purpose of closing the excretion filter so that water can be withheld to give the organism a chance to survive. The instant activation of this water retention program is vital because, ***without water, all metabolic processes stop functioning.***

Hello, slow metabolism!

With this in mind, let's take a deeper dive into the AIRE model.

**ABANDONMENT** conflicts are all about being left behind, deserted, discarded, banished, undesired, and even ostracized. We may be separated, neglected, passed over, and, of course, abandoned.

Those experiencing abandonment may feel cut off from a source of emotional or other sustenance that has been withdrawn. Abandonment need not be physical. We all know a parent or individual who has emotionally withdrawn their love. A classic example is the newborn being shuttled away from Mom within seconds of life so the doctors and workers can perform the requisite measurements and evaluations. Another example would be the child coming home from school only to find out that one parent has left the nest due to a divorce.

**ISOLATION** conflicts are quite similar to abandonment and are all about feeling alone and emotionally unsupported. You're on your own, with no one to lean on, no one to hold you up, no support, total seclusion.

As we get older and our parents pass away, kids move away, and friends come and go, we tend to feel isolated more than at any time in our lives. The mobile society of the 21st century is where we no longer establish roots and strong ties. The extended family is so often a thing of the past. Hospitalization can also isolate us. Simply having our own approach as to how we choose to address our health issues can be isolating. At times we can feel like the black sheep. With the increased incidence of bullying, cyberbullying, and social isolation, children are often left to deal with these difficult social dynamics alone. Technologically, we are more connected than at any previous time in our history, yet so very alone. A friend of mine has over three hundred thousand Instagram followers yet lacks true personal and emotional support.

A **REFUGEE** conflict is all about feeling like we are without roots, without a home, without a nest, out of place, out of familiar surroundings, and out of our element.

Before I learned about the KCT conflict, I noticed that when I traveled, I would always wake up with bloating and constipation for several days. I had always attributed this to irregular routines associated with traveling. I came to understand that traveling for me was a track that reopened a refugee or water retention conflict. As soon as I arrived home, the bloating and constipation would recede. I was working with a woman months back that swore she had no refugee conflict until we discovered that her family had moved 22 times in her 34 years! This poor woman was a gypsy without a home.

An **EXISTENCE** conflict arises when we feel our very life, even our livelihood, is threatened – by a diagnosis, a near miss relative to an accident, a loss of job or career, or loss of a home to foreclosure, which also has links to refugee conflict.

Our existence can also be threatened by fluid (moldy, water-damaged buildings) and/or money. It can also be threatened by bankruptcy, enormous credit card debt, and or failing economic support (money is liquidity.) Think about it... drowning in debt, staying above water, and liquidating one's savings bonds. It's about losing everything–our existence and our livelihoods are at stake. Our existence can also be threatened by alcoholism. This falls under our safety being threatened by water, or fluid. We may also feel abandoned and isolated by the alcoholic family upbringing.

The obesity epidemic is due, in part, to the chronicity of this AIRE program. Two liters of water in our tissue weighs four and a half pounds. We can retain upwards of ten times that when both kidneys are active with conflict. Of course, we need to account for other possibilities, such as diet, exercise, and additional biological conflicts, such as the thyroid. This is weight that will not come off through proper diet, exercise, or supplementation. It is an evolutionary survival program expressing itself. It will not change until the psyche is able to release the conflict and all tracks. Upon release, the kidney collecting tubules will "loosen," and the water will be pressed out from the body level as well as from the cerebral level as the urinary or pee-pee phase begins.

### *INFLAMED GUT*

Finally, the Inflamed Gut, also sometimes referenced the "Brain Gut," is a byproduct of overwhelm. An inflamed gut is the body's way of saying, "May Day! May Day!" Stress levels are high, burning like a fiery furnace, resulting in inflammation in different organs and tissues.

Anxiety and migraines result from a "danger and powerlessness conflict"—feeling like you can't control a situation. Heart disease is an "overwhelmed conflict," brought on by negative stress overload, while arthritis is an overwhelming "self devaluation conflict," often stemming from humiliation, comparing yourself to others, or believing you're not good enough.

The body keeps the score.

*Identify your Gut Type! Find details for the 5 Gut Types Quiz in the Resources section at the back of this book. You can also map out any potential Gut-Brain "conflicts" or stressors driving your symptoms using the Gut-Brain Connection Cheat Sheet.*

*What if you don't have symptoms at all?*

Congratulations! You may be one of the rare people who have the "Golden Gut"—a healthy, balanced biome. You experience daily, well-formed bowel movements (1-3 times per day); you have no bloating or gas after meals or food intolerances; you don't *need* coffee or sugar to function; you're rarely sick or rundown; you maintain regular exercise and good sleep hygiene; and you eat a nutrient-dense, varied diet. Overall, you listen to your body, and you are intuitive.

## ASSESSMENT 2: HEALTH STORY TIMELINE.

Your Health Story is a critical step for identifying the root causes behind any health or gut challenges you may be experiencing. Feeling unwell does not happen overnight, and as you improve your understanding and identify the pieces of your Health Story, the stressors, life circumstances, and triggers that have led you to where you are today, the better you are able to move in a *new* direction and establish answers as to the *why's* behind how you feel.

## ***EXHIBIT A:* CATCHING A COLD**

Catching a cold is a great example of a perfect storm, health-wise. Catching a cold does not suddenly happen on its own. Although you may wake up one day and feel under the weather, chances are there were a handful of triggers that led you there, including:

- Running off of five to six hours of sleep for multiple nights in a row;
- Not drinking enough water;
- Exposure to the cold bugs at work or school;
- Eating more sugar than usual;
- Overworked (overtraining, overcommitting, being overzealous with work deadlines);
- Not taking your probiotics;
- A "stink" conflict.

Multiple triggers and stressors work together to create the perfect storm for SIBO, candida, Lyme disease, asthma, infertility, fatigue, high cholesterol, cancer, and beyond. Many triggers and stressors date back weeks, months, and years prior to a health decline or diagnosis—even as far back as your birth and childhood.

Your Health Story helps you think through and detail your health history as well as plot it chronologically, often revealing various factors and identifying triggers that have led your health to where you are today. Your Health Story includes your birth story, predisposing factors, triggering events, and ongoing stressors—all factors that shape your health for the worse or better.

# YOUR BIRTH STORY.

The first two years of life are the most crucial in microbiome development. I hate to break it to you, but the cards were stacked against you early if you were:

- Delivered via cesarean section;
- Fed formula;
- Given antibiotics.

Trust me; I can relate. I'm three for three on that list. Even if you only experienced one or two of these, your gut health took a hit, but if you're like me, you're what I call a "triple threat." Life and the circumstances of our formative years thwarted our gut bacteria formation from the very start during our most formidable period. For example, breast milk contains over seven different bacterial species essential for seeding a child's gut, whereas formulas contain a big whopping...zero.

Newborns delivered by c-sections tend to lack strains of gut bacteria found in healthy children and adults. Instead, the guts of C-section babies are dominated by gram-negative bacteria that circulate in hospitals. Your microbial fingerprint sticks with you for a lifetime, and stool samples of adults *still* reflect the same microbiome they had as babies and help researchers determine whether or not you were delivered by C-section or vaginal birth.

Other considerations that also play a role include the foods your mom ate when she was pregnant with you and *her* microbiome health, in addition to any childhood traumas you experienced in early life, big or small. A Columbia University study comparing children adopted from orphanages or foster care on or before approximately they were two years old to children raised by a biological caregiver found that children with past caregiving disruptions showed higher levels of symptoms that included stomach aches, constipation, vomiting, and nausea. The children with a history of early caregiving disruptions also had distinctly different gut microbiomes from those raised with biological caregivers from birth. Brain scans showed that the children raised by parents had increased gut microbiome diversity, which is linked to the prefrontal cortex, a region of the brain known to help regulate emotions. This confirmed other research that has demonstrated that a history of trauma or abuse has been reported in up to half of adults with (IBS), at a prevalence twice that of patients without IBS.

The word "trauma" may invoke images of car crashes and the loss of a loved one. However, trauma also includes experiences that you may easily block out or discount as "traumatic," such as being left out or picked on at school, hearing frequent, intense arguments between your parents, an eating disorder that started in your teens, emotional abuse or neglect, financial strain in your family, or a bicycle or sporting accident. I simply call these "conflict shocks"—stressors that catch us off guard, leave us feeling out of control, or that we don't have the resources or strategies to process or deal with them.

Generational traumas may also be passed down through your family and left unaddressed, like addiction, poverty, or illness. For example, my great-great-grandparents were Holocaust survivors. My grandfather and dad were ridiculed and beaten for being Jewish. My mom was adopted and raised in a broken marriage home. My "ancestors" and predecessors were resilient *and* also carried many emotions of anxiety, fear, anger, and sadness etched in their DNA that was passed down to me. Our issues can get locked into our tissues until we become aware and start to resolve them.

## *PREDISPOSING FACTORS:*

These are the factors, genetic or acquired, that predispose you to a health imbalance or pattern of disease. Imbalance does not happen overnight, and it's often the slow build-up over time that can result in the onset of ill health. It could be due to growing up in a home where home-cooked meals meant frozen chicken nuggets and French fries, taking birth control for five years—a common precursor to SIBO; or having the MTHFR or HLA-DQ genes, which contribute to poor detoxification or suppressed immune function respectively.

## *TRIGGERING EVENTS:*

These can be events, circumstances, or stressors that directly provoke the symptoms and signs of illness. For instance, getting bitten by a tick in the case of Lyme disease, living in a moldy rental home and ending up with fungal and mold overgrowth in your body, or food poisoning from bad Chinese takeout that sparked IBS.

## *ONGOING STRESSORS:*

Ongoing stressors are lifestyle, nutritional, medication, and mental/emotional factors that do not contribute to your personal body balance or wellness. It's important to note that some of these stressors may be perfectly healthy for some, but the methods or ways in which you engage in them are not ideal for you. Examples include intermittent fasting when your body is already experiencing HPA-axis dysfunction; overtraining; accidental under-eating on a low-carb diet; sleeping for only five to six hours most nights; staring at screens and blue lights for eight plus hours per day, and drinking three cups of coffee per day.

### *GUT-BRAIN CONFLICTS:*

At a deeper level beyond physical stressors, are there any significant emotional stressors or conflict "shocks" that have occurred in your life preceding the onset of your health issues? Put them on your timeline.

Gut-Brain Check Questions
Use the following questions to dig deeper:

- Was there a time when you heard something or saw something you could not "digest" but you had to, or when you were afraid for survival? (Morsel conflict)
- Was there a time when someone was having a serious go at you, and you had to protect yourself? (Attack conflict)
- Was there a time when someone said something to you, even though you knew it was wrong, and you let them get away with it, but it devastated your self-esteem? Or, has such an instance left you feeling worthless or when your self-esteem was shattered? (Self-devaluation/esteem conflict)
- Was there a time when you were left all alone to fend for yourself and you were abandoned? (Territory conflict)
- Was there a time when someone was trying to take something or someone away from you where you wanted to fight them or run away from them but could not? (Territory/separation)

# ASSESSMENT 3: THE GUT CHECK METHOD

How do you feel?

The answer to that question may be what led you to pick up this book in the first place. Bloated? Constipated? Tired? Brain foggy? Heavy? You fill in the blank. Regardless of your symptoms, there is no doubt that how we feel impacts our total quality of life.

*How you feel* also points to an even bigger question: ***Why do you feel this way?***

## SPINACH EATING SAM

Popeye the Sailor Man would have been proud: At least three times per day, Sam ate something green. Typically spinach. Sauteed. Steamed. As part of a raw leafy salad. In smoothies. In soups.

He did this until the day he ran out of spinach and was forced to substitute his usual morning greens with something else—leftover arugula in his breakfast smoothie and some romaine lettuce with lunch instead of spinach salad.

Surprisingly, no brain fog or IBS symptoms that day. Long story short, Sam's accidental spinach food intolerance test led him to uncover a deep-rooted histamine intolerance that he had been experiencing for years.

Spinach is not innately bad. However, if you have histamine intolerance, as Sam did, then eating spinach three times per day is not great.

The clincher? Sam *never* would have uncovered spinach as one of the drivers behind his daily symptoms without being able to suddenly recognize how his body felt.

So I'll ask again: How do *you* feel?

The answer is exactly what Assessment 3 is all about—connecting to the wisdom in your body and your gut intuition. Connecting to the wisdom in your body or your gut intuition is a skill hardwired in you. You were born knowing exactly what your body needed and what it was saying. As a baby, you cried when you were hungry, turned your head away when you were full, slept when you felt tired, and laughed when you were full of joy. You listened to your gut intuition.

The sensations we feel in our body offer important messages about our health, stress levels, and relationships. You may find that your heart feels lighter in the presence of someone you care about, or maybe you get butterflies in your stomach when you're feeling anxious. Even hunger or tiredness can clue us into the fact that we need to engage in more self-care. These signals might seem very basic, but in our over-stimulated, head-centered society, it's very easy to lose touch with them and consequently very easy to lose touch with the reasons why our health goes south in the first place.

Intuitiveness simply means listening to your body and eating and living accordingly to its physical needs and cues. For example, intuitive eating is eating when you are hungry and stopping when you are full. It is eating a steak when your body needs iron energy; sipping bone broth and ginger tea when you feel sick; intuitively craving watermelon on a hot summer day, and not eating the same foods or doing the same exact workouts every day. Intuitively, your body wants variety.

Unfortunately, gut intuition is often the first naturally born skill to go in modern-day society, especially if you have a history that's anything like this:

- Lacking local and seasonal foods in your diet;
- Consuming processed foods or fake "health" foods that disrupts your gut microbiome and warps your tastebuds, such as artificially sweetened waters and yogurt, cardboard-like protein bars, and imitation keto-friendly Cheetos;
- Eating the same things every day;
- Emotionally eating when you have a bad day;
- Circadian rhythm disruption, from late night eating to eating six small meals, forced intermittent fasting, and dieting.

Retraining ourselves to be mindful can help reset our eating and lifestyle habits. Mindfulness occurs when we are present and consciously aware of thoughts, feelings, bodily sensations, our body's needs, and our surrounding environment without judgment or without necessarily acting upon our first instincts.

In terms of eating, mindful eating uses the power of our mental abilities to help us determine what's best for our body's needs and health. For example, mindful eating is eating one cookie instead of 12, knowing that while your taste buds may crave sugar, a little bit goes a long way. Mindful eating is eating turkey sausage instead of eggs in the morning because you realize eggs make you feel nauseous or opting for coconut milk over cow's milk because your skin breaks out every time you consume dairy products. Mindful eating is not forcing yourself to eat a salad or a dry chicken breast and broccoli because you should, although mindful eating is sometimes eating—even if you don't feel like it—because you know your body needs enough fuel to support its hormone balance, energy levels, and your workouts.

You get the picture: intuitive eating and living are eating and living based on your body's innate wiring and cues; mindful eating plays back up, helping you decipher how your body feels when you eat certain foods and determining what foods make you feel best.

Connecting to the wisdom in your body does not happen overnight but is something you can practice. One of the simplest ways I've found to do this is something I call the "Gut Check Method." Whenever something is "off" in how you feel, or you're trying to figure out what your gut wants and needs, your *first* approach should be to ask these three questions:

1. What do I feel?
2. Why do I feel this way?
3. What do I need?

For example:

1. What do I feel? A headache.
2. Why do I feel this way? I only drank one cup of water today and missed protein with breakfast.
3. What do I need? More water and some bone broth could hit the spot right now.

Or one more:

1. What do I feel? Constipated. I didn't poop today.
2. Why do I feel this way? I missed out on fiber with my dinner last night, and I only slept five hours instead of my usual seven. My body is off its rhythm.
3. What do I need? Some "poo" supports (like digestive bitters and magnesium), deep breathing, and better sleep tonight should help things get back on track.

## 8 GUT LOVE SUPERPOWERS

More often than not, the answer behind why we feel "off" in the first place is found somewhere in us being out of touch with our body and out of touch with our intuition, especially the eight essentials that I call the "8 Gut Love Superpowers":

1. **Breath**—Are you breathing well and oxygenating your tissues appropriately?
2. **Hydration**—Are you drinking enough water?

3. **Digestion**—Are you chewing your food really well? Do you have enough enzymes and stomach acid?
4. **Nutrients**—Are you eating gut-loving foods?
5. **Sleep**—Are you getting deep sleep—6-9 hours most nights?
6. **Movement**—Moving daily, whether you have seven minutes or sixty, and not too much?
7. **Detox**—Is your body able to clear out toxins? Are you pooping and sweating regularly? Avoiding toxic chemicals in products, foods, and environmental exposures?
8. **Connection**—Do you have social connections? Are you connected to your passions, doing things you love and enjoy?

It's the little everyday lifestyle things that make a *big* difference in how we feel. If listening to your body sounds impossible now, start with Assessment 3— doing a "Gut Check" by keeping a three-day Food, Mood, and Poo Log.

In this log, you'll not only log precisely what you eat, but you'll also record how you feel *before* and *after* meals, including your level of hunger and fullness, your daily poo (time and texture), and other influential lifestyle factors such as how many hours you slept the night before, the type of movement you did that day, and your water, supplements, and caffeine intake.

Given the fact that what we eat, what we digest, and our lifestyle habits hold the greatest impact on how we feel on a daily basis, by cultivating our awareness of these factors, we can better understand what may be driving symptoms or flares.

***Connect to your gut:*** *Keep a* ***3-Day Food, Mood, and Poo Log*** *(in the Resources section at the back of this book) to begin raising awareness for how your food, daily routines, and lifestyle habits affect how you feel.*

# BONUS: FOOD INTOLERANCE EXPERIMENTS

Do you have food intolerances? Now it's time to analyze your log to assess for any digestive difficulties, triggers, or red flags that may explain more about how you feel.

We are what we eat. Rephrase: Our gut biome is what we eat. Food is one of the most telling signs of what types of gut issues we are dealing with underneath the hood.

For example, feel sick, gassy, or burpy after eating fattier foods—even healthy fats like salmon, avocado, or butter? You may have a congested gallbladder. Do proteins feel like a rock in your stomach? Stomach acid deficiency. Super bloated—no matter what you eat, but especially when you eat FODMAP foods, like Brussels sprouts, apples, or yogurt? SIBO—small intestinal bacterial overgrowth—is super common. Can't tolerate peanuts, eggs, or dairy? Leaky gut and autoimmunity.

Sure, we certainly can all agree that certain foods are not ideal for most human microbiomes, like processed foods, industrial seed oils, and refined sugar. However, there are hundreds of other foods that fall into a "gray" area, meaning some foods trigger food sensitivity symptoms for some people but not others. Apples can make one person feel super bloated; another person immediately has to run to the bathroom if they eat sweet potatoes. Another seems to tolerate sourdough bread or rice just fine, while the other gets brain fog instantly when they eat carbs. How do food intolerances happen, even to healthy foods? Your gut bacteria *and* your Gut-Brain Connection have something to do with it.

For one, if you have dysbiosis (gut bacteria imbalances) or impaired digestive mechanics, loss of "oral tolerance" is quite common, which is the loss of your ability to tolerate a variety of foods due to reduced variety of gut bacteria, enzymes, gallbladder function or stomach acid to digest those foods.

As for the Gut-Brain Connection, remember back to little Nick, who developed an intolerance to his beloved peanut butter and jelly sandwich around the same time his parents split, or Bacon Intolerance Becky, who developed an intolerance to bacon around the same time she found out her husband was cheating on her while she was cooking bacon? The brain—specifically the "limbic system" has a tendency to associate certain foods with certain stressors if the "perfect storm" happens.

My former sensitivities to histamine-rich foods, oxalates, and "healthy" foods like sweet potatoes, grass-fed beef, nuts, eggs, apples, broccoli, and beyond also are a great example of how food sensitivity happens with stress. When I got sick with mold (a huge stressor), I became sensitive to multiple foods that the body associated with stress, both due to mold and my history of anorexia. When I had anorexia, my brain thought sweet potatoes had too many carbs, beef and nuts were too high in fat, and apples, broccoli, and egg whites were "safe" foods—both fear foods and diet foods were associated with stress.

Boom! Food sensitivities galore when significant "indigestible" stress struck later in life! My brain and body went right back to the "old days" and said, "Nope! Not into these foods!" This, however, changed when I began to take back my "power" and learned how to heal my food sensitivities naturally.

Similarly, another client of mine found herself with food sensitivities to "everything!" This occurred during her seven-year battle with autoimmune disease, mold exposure, hormone imbalances, and gut issues galore. When we met, she was only eating about five to ten foods because that was all she could tolerate.

Why did this happen? Deep down, this client had a deep-seated belief that certain foods would make her fat, a belief which began at age 14 when her dad told her "carbs are bad." Enter: Stress in her life, which correlated stress with food fears too.

The good news: You can improve your food tolerance! And, instead of spending money on a non-validated food intolerance test marketed to you on social media, give these three Food Intolerance Experiments a try first.

## *EXPERIMENT 1:* FOOD INTOLERANCE TIMELINE

Got food intolerances? Do the Gut-Brain "work" to identify the *root cause* or "indigestible" conflict(s) associated with your food intolerance.

Ask yourself: What stressors are associated with this food (example: "I used to carefully count out almonds and restrict my calories; or I told myself carbs are bad")? Can you recall any specific conflict or indigestible stress in your life around the time you consumed this food? Often, clients recall simply being told certain foods are "bad" for them or seeing the results of a food intolerance test as seeding the belief that they cannot eat that food ever again.

Also, recognize the correlation between eating certain foods or trying new foods and stress or fears in your life today. Think back to the milkshake study discussed in Chapter 3. Remember, we are the stories we tell ourselves, and our mindset plays a huge role in how our body responds to food or not.

## *EXPERIMENT 2:* **FOOD SWAP CHALLENGE.**

***Step 1: Identify your top five foods:***

Look at your three-day Food, Mood, and Poo Log and determine which foods you eat most frequently. Since our gut bacteria often crave foods we are intolerant to, and dysbiosis can also be a byproduct of eating the *same foods* every day, make a list of the top five foods you eat on a daily basis. Note: These foods may not even be sugar or items from McDonald's. Your top five foods may include foods you consider healthy, such as broccoli, ground turkey, almonds, bananas, and the coffee you consume every morning. Any food that you find yourself eating every day should go on your list.

***Step 2: Replace your top five listed foods for three to seven days:***

After determining what you're eating most frequently, replace your top five foods with five different foods for the next three to seven days. For example, you might try asparagus instead of broccoli, ground bison or shredded chicken instead of ground turkey, tiger nuts instead of almonds, blueberries instead of bananas, and green tea instead of coffee. By doing so, you'll be better able to determine if your daily symptoms are simply a by-product of the foods you're eating, a digestive dysfunction, or something else.

***Step 3: Observe:***

Observe how you feel for the next three days. Include your mental as well as your physical states, and note such things as the length and quality of your sleep and your levels of energy and fatigue during the day.

***Step 4: Reintroduce:***

Reintroduce your old favorite foods, one day at a time and for a period of 24 hours. Note how you feel, the positives and/or negatives.

***Step 5: Gut-Brain Check:***

If you identify any food intolerances from these experiments, do the Gut-Brain "work." Can you recall any specific stressor or time in your life around this food? Resolution often comes with awareness of the root cause conflicts that preceded disease *and* proactive deciding that you choose to increase your food tolerance.

## EXPERIMENT 3: DIGESTIVE SUPERPOWERS.

Different types of foods require different types of digestive functions and supports like enzymes to break them down. If we have a "weak link" in our digestion, we will typically experience elevated symptoms when that type of food is consumed, such as bloating after eating a sweet potato if you have SIBO and/or a pancreatic enzyme production deficiency. Observe how you feel with the following foods eaten alone:

- Food: Complete animal protein source (chicken, beef, turkey).
  What it may mean if you don't feel well: Low stomach acid.
- Food: Healthy fat (fish, fish oil, ghee, avocado, butter).
  What it may mean if you don't feel well: Gallbladder congestion.
- Food: FODMAP foods (Brussels sprouts, broccoli, cauliflower, onion, garlic, etc.).
  What it may mean if you don't feel well: Dysbiosis, SIBO, candida, and/or poor gallbladder function.
- Food: Histamine-rich food (spinach, canned wild salmon or tuna, fermented foods).
  What it may mean if you don't feel well: immune gut, metabolic endotoxemia, SIBO, candida
- Food: Lectin-containing foods (beans, peanuts, lentils, tomatoes, potatoes, eggplant, fruits, wheat, and other grains).
  What it may mean if you don't feel well: immune gut, metabolic endotoxemia.
- Food: Carb challenge (starchy tuber, like a sweet potato or butternut squash).
  What it may mean if you don't feel well: dysbiosis, bacterial overgrowth, and/or digestive enzyme deficiencies.

# ASSESSMENT 4: THE GOLDEN POO CHALLENGE

The average American's morning is *not* complete without coffee. However, my morning is not complete without a Golden Poo. You know, that euphoric feeling of complete elimination that makes you do the "poo dance" (sort of like your dog that runs in circles after going for a number 2 or your baby that smiles and laughs after filling their diaper).

Your poo patterns say a lot about the health of your gut. Just like a "regular menstrual cycle" or "regular blood pressure," your poo patterns are your daily report card for good health. So, what exactly is the "Golden Poo"?

Poop, or feces, is a mixture of 75% water and dead bacteria that helps us digest our food. Normal, healthy poo is fully formed, light brown, and sausage-shaped in an "S" or "C," about three to five inches long, and leaves you with the feeling of complete, full elimination. Sometimes it can be green or red if you eat green veggies or beets—as long as it's not loose and watery. It's also okay if it's a little smelly—just not foul.

Ideally, if you are eating three balanced meals per day, a squeaky clean digestive system would have you pooping anywhere from 1-3 times a day of normally formed stools and feeling completely eliminated (not hard to pass, loose or watery, or bits and pieces). You will also experience ideal bowel transit time, which is the amount of time it takes for the food we eat to pass through our digestive system and get poo-ed out should be between 12 to 24 hours.

If you experience anything other than the aforementioned, Golden Poo may not be on your side.

Loose, watery stools mean you're not digesting something appropriately, especially if there is a fast transit time. Loose, watery stools can also mean you have SIBO, a gut infection, low stomach acid, or an "indigestible conflict" in your life. Likewise, if your poop is loose, something is *off*.

Dehydration and low minerals help you absorb your water—especially magnesium, sodium, and potassium bicarbonate. Are you drinking enough water *with* minerals? If you feel thirsty ever during the day, the answer is a clear-cut *no.*

Brain-Gut stress and gallbladder congestion are two other really common conundrums that cause constipation. The vagus nerve that connects the gut and brain also helps push poop through your system. If your body is highly stressed, then the vagus nerve locks up, and poo motility slows down. As for your gallbladder, this small but mighty organ releases bile when you eat—a sludge-like liquid that digests toxins and nutrients and also acts like a natural laxative for healthy bowel movements. Bile softens stool and speeds up how fast it moves through the colon. Gallbladder problems are one of the most overlooked problems of bloating and constipation.

**Golden Poo Challenge:** What does your poo say about you? Take the Golden Poo Challenge. Use your Gut Check 3 Day Food, Mood, and Poo Log to keep a record of your daily poo patterns—when you go, what it looks like, identify any "causes" of your poo, and use the Golden Poo Chart as a guide.

# ASSESSMENT 5: CLINICAL LAB TESTS

Beyond self-assessment, clinical lab testing can be an adjunctive "health detective" strategy for "tuning in" to your gut.

When properly used and interpreted correctly, clinical lab testing is like turning bright lights on in a dark room, or hitting the dart board with your eyes open instead of shooting darts, blindfolded, with anti-candida diets, Whole30 repeats, methylation supplements, and tummy shrinking waistbands dig a bit deeper for any underlying pathologies.

## *10 COMMON GUT PATHOLOGIES*

Gut problems go far beyond bloating or IBS. Here are ten common gut pathologies (underlying imbalances) that may arise from gut imbalances. Unfortunately, many gastroenterologists (*and* integrative or functional medicine doctors, for that matter may not screen for these *or* may inaccurately diagnose you (Note: This is *not* an exhaustive list).

1. Autoimmune gut;
2. Fungal overgrowth;
3. Dysbiosis
4. Gut infections (parasites, viruses, and bacterial infections);
5. Hormone and thyroid imbalances;
6. Leaky gut or metabolic endotoxemia;
7. Liver, gallbladder, or pancreatic dysfunction (low enzyme and bile production);

8. Low stomach acid and gastric conditions;
9. SIBO (Small Intestinal Bacterial Overgrowth);
10. Dis-Ease or significant emotional stress.

How do you know if you have any of these? Don't worry about the details. This is where working with a skilled clinician or joining the Total Gut Reset program can come into play to help you navigate the Wild Wild West of gut health.

Before we discuss the top clinical tests for a Total Gut Reset, let's set the record straight: there are *tons* of lab tests on the market, with more becoming readily available directly to consumers. From stool tests to genetic screenings, hormone panels, food intolerance kits, and adrenal fatigue hacking, lab testing is often touted as a panacea for taking back your health. However, while testing *can* offer valuable health insights, it's vital to realize that, just like probiotics or your ideal diet, not *all* testing is created equal.

Similar to how no two burgers are created equal (there is a difference between a McDonald's Big Mac with Grade D meat and a homemade, grass-fed beef burger), no two stool tests, food intolerance tests, hormone tests, or heavy metals tests are created equal either—especially from third party lab companies. Moreover, not all lab tests are beneficial, meaning, yes, you *can* test your stool, blood, spit, or urine and receive results, but do those results actually provide clinically relevant, valuable information that will help you improve your health?

Not always.

I'll be brutally honest: Sometimes, I think it's easier to win the lottery than to get the proper tests you need. Even if you do get the proper tests ordered, it can be a nightmare to find someone qualified to help you interpret the results. Not only that, but ordering the wrong tests is like lighting several hundred dollar bills on fire. Unfortunately, many commercial companies and healthcare practitioners are unaware of the differences in testing types and methods, often resulting in both unnecessary treatments and an over-reliance on testing methods that may not be entirely accurate or beneficial.

## *HOW DO YOU KNOW WHAT FUNCTIONAL LAB TESTS YOU NEED?*

So, is lab testing really worth it? And, if so, which tests should you do?

It's important to keep in mind that just because a lab company promotes a test with studies to back it up or claims you'll discover tons of information with which to hack your health, that does not mean it's true.

For instance: Food intolerance testing may tell you you're sensitive to apples, almonds, and broccoli, but is this because you eat these foods every day and you have more of these circulating food proteins in your body already, or because you really can't eat them? And just because your 23&Me says you have an MTHFR variation in your genes (like 50 percent of the population), does it mean you need to take methylated B-12 and folate supplements, or that instead you should focus on optimizing your epigenetics to influence your genes (your gut health, air quality, nutrition)?

When in doubt, the number one thing I consider when trying to determine if a certain test is the right option is this: Will the results of the test change the treatment protocol? The answer to that question helps to instantly rule out unnecessary testing. Generally, in terms of testing, *less* is more.

Although there are tons of tests you *can* run that may be beneficial, I prefer to start as *lean* as possible and add additional testing if needed.

The tests you do need form a triple threat:

1. Functional blood chemistry panel (CBC, metabolic panel, lipid panel, iron panel, complete thyroid and hormone panel, Vitamin D);
2. Gut microbiome testing: Comprehensive stool analysis;
3. Optional wild card: Specific to *you:*
    - Hair or serum mineral analysis;
    - SIBO breath testing;
    - Saliva and urine hormone cortisol testing;
    - Gluten-intolerance and gluten cross-reactivity testing (bloodwork, Cyrex Array 3 and/or 4);
    - Mold/mycotoxin testing (urine and blood work markers);

The reason my number three top test is a wild card is to allow for a little more specificity for each patient, depending on the primary symptoms and chief complaints they come to me with. For example, suppose you're experiencing bloating after every meal and alternating stool consistency. In that case, a SIBO breath test may be a beneficial addition to your testing lineup, whereas if you present with symptoms of mold or mycotoxin illness such as fatigue, brain fog, or histamine intolerance, a mold/mycotoxin urine test would make sense. We may not even need to run a wild card test at all.

If, after running these initial tests, you find you're still hitting ceilings, that is when follow-up testing comes into play.

## *DON'T GO IT ALONE*

One of the most important steps for running lab tests and addressing findings appropriately is to work with a skilled practitioner. You can use the best testing methods and find out the most information in the world, but if you choose the wrong practitioner, you probably *won't* get the proper therapeutic program.

I recommend working with a practitioner who practices and regularly studies Functional Medicine—a scope of practice utilized by some medical doctors, osteopathic doctors, and allied health providers (nutritionists, dietitians, therapists, and health coaches). These specially trained practitioners aim to help patients identify the root cause(s) of chronic, lingering, or apparently unsolvable health issues and to help prevent disease and optimize your health—not just address symptoms. You want a practitioner who focuses on *fully* understanding your health history (not just your immediate health history) and the lifestyle factors (nutrition, supplements, sleep, exercise) that contribute to both wellness and disease. You also want a practitioner who doesn't run every test under the sun or prescribe supplements or programs with little guidance. Look for a practitioner through a reputably trained program (or several).

# GUT CHECK POINT

Test, don't guess, to better customize the foods, supplements, and lifestyle hacks for *you*.

## REFERENCES


1. R. Cabrera-Rubio, M. C. Collado, K. Laitinen, S. Salminen, E. Isolauri, A. Mira. The human milk microbiome changes over lactation and is shaped by maternal weight and mode of delivery. *American Journal of Clinical Nutrition*, 2012; 96 (3): 544 DOI: 10.3945/ajcn.112.037382
2. Shao, Y. *et al. Nature* https://doi.org/10.1038/s41586-019-1560-1 (2019).
3. Callaghan, B. L., Fields, A., Gee, D. G., Gabard-Durnam, L., Caldera, C., Humphreys, K. L., ... Tottenham, N. (undefined/ed). Mind and gut: Associations between mood and gastrointestinal distress in children exposed to adversity. Development and Psychopathology, 1–20. https://doi.org/10.1017/S0954579419000087
4. Videlock EJ, Adeyemo M, Licudine A, *et al.* Childhood trauma is associated with hypothalamic-pituitary-adrenal axis responsiveness in irritable bowel syndrome. *Gastroenterology*. 2009;137(6):1954-1962. doi:10.1053/j.gastro.2009.08.058

# PART THREE: TAKING CARE AND CONTROL

# CHAPTER 10:
# STEP TWO–EIGHT GUT-LOVE SUPERPOWERS

Everybody loves a good underdog story.

David, a scrawny shepherd boy, defeats seven-foot giant Goliath with nothing but a slingshot.

Cinderella, the "peasant" princess under the thumb of her evil stepmother, meets Prince Charming and rises from rags to riches.

Elizabeth Smart is kidnapped at age 14 from her home and goes missing for nine months. Smart goes on to become an advocate for missing persons and victims of sexual assault.

Teen surfer Bethany Hamilton loses her arm to a shark and courageously overcomes all odds to become a champion again.

Harry Potter, an orphan, living with his abusive aunt and uncle and their bully son in a closet under the staircase, discovers he is a wizard with incredible superpowers.

And after all hope is lost, Dorothy discovers she also has the power *inside herself* to go back home to Kansas after a long, winding journey on the Yellow Brick Road.

Well, love to break it to you, my friend: You hold inside *yourself* a great "underdog story" to up-level how you look, move, feel, think, and poo, Eight Gut-Love Superpowers, to be exact, that comprise the essence of Step Two in your Total Gut Reset: Take care of your gut.

# TAKE CARE OF YOUR GUT

One of my favorite questions to ask my patients after we have worked together is: *What helped you the most during our work together?*

Very rarely do they say a restrictive elimination diet, expensive lab test finding, or supplement. More often than not, that answer has something to do with a simple daily lifestyle hack and less stress in their lives.

## *EXHIBIT A:* TIFFANY TAKES ON TURKEY DAY

"Dr. Lauryn, you're *never* going to believe it! I went home for Thanksgiving and ate stuffing and corn casserole and pumpkin pie—things I have not eaten in years, and I didn't react!"

This news brought tears to my eyes. Just six months earlier, Tanya was singing a different tune. Literally. The budding famous jazz singer was completely sidelined from the career that she loved and feeling both depleted and depleted.

Diagnosed with toxic mold illness, Lyme disease, Bartonella, fluoroquinolone toxicity, SIBO, parasites, and mast cell activation syndrome; when I first met Tanya, her chart contained nine lives worth of lab test results and treatment protocols, and this history was less than one year old. To top it off, Tiffany was eating only five to ten foods and reacting to almost every building or home she went into with brain fog, skin rashes, and IBS. Fast forward to learning how to take care of her gut and trust her gut, and it was as if amnesia had happened in her body. Her body was now ready to be well and leave sickness behind.

* * *

The health journey is a marathon, not a sprint. We are in it for the long haul, and although perfect health may not exist, better health does.

Sometimes on the mission to improve your health, it's easy to want to try to take the wheel—chug more green juice, order ten supplements, cut out more carbs, turn to Dr. Google, and work out for two hours every day, when all your body needs is *balance*.

I call this balance your *baseline*. Your baseline consists of eight essentials that I call your eight gut reset superpowers. They're what your body needs to feel good without drastic measures. These eight essentials, or as I prefer to call them, Superpowers, are:

1. Breath
2. Hydration;
3. Absorption;
4. Nutrients
5. Rest
6. Movement
7. Detox
8. Connection

Before even thinking about extreme dieting or ordering boatloads of supplements, are you optimizing your gut reset superpowers? Answer "yes" or "no" to the following questions.

## BASELINE GUT CHECK-IN

1. Am I breathing properly and making space for "breath breaks" or "recess breaks" in my day?
2. Am I drinking half my body weight in ounces of clean water daily?
3. Am I chewing my food well, and do I have optimal stomach acid, digestive enzymes, and bacteria for proper nutrient absorption?
4. Am I eating a varied, fiber-rich, nutrient-dense diet?
5. Am I getting six to nine hours of unbroken, quality sleep and proper light exposure at the right times of the day?
6. Am I moving daily—but not overtraining?
7. Am I pooping and sweating daily and avoiding unnecessary toxic exposures?
8. Do I have a connection to people and spirituality? Am I doing things I love—my passions, my purpose?

Above all: whenever something is off in the health department, your first approach should be to ask *why?*

*Why do I feel bloated or constipated? Why is my skin breaking out? Why do I have a headache? Why are my allergies flaring? Why am I more anxious than usual?*

Once you ask yourself *why*, you can then conduct a self-assessment of where your lifestyle, nutrition, and gut health align in comparison to your baseline, your Eight Gut Love Superpowers for feeling good. More often than not, the answer lies somewhere in a lack of balance in our baseline.

Remember: When given the right tools, your body innately wants to heal itself. And the cool thing is these eight habits have never gone out of style. Unlike the latest debate over whether no carb, high protein, or non-protein are the answer or the latest Taebo, then Orange Theory, then Barry's Bootcamp craze, these eight habits have stood the test of time for centuries.

Without further ado, let's dissect each of the Eight Gut Love Superpowers that will help you achieve your Total Gut Reset. As a bonus, I will also provide you with an actionable Gut Love Habit for each of the Superpowers, making them even easier to adopt.

This is where the magic happens. The best part? When you unleash the Eight Superpowers together, you may find that you don't require any other further testing, diets, or supplements at all.

# CHAPTER 11: SUPERPOWER 1: BREATH

***In case of emergency, oxygen masks will drop down in front of you. Please pull the mask down toward your face and place the mask over your mouth and nose. If you are traveling with a child, please attend to yourself first, then the child.***
***- Federal Aviation Regulations***

## THE ELEPHANT IN THE ROOM: OXIDATIVE STRESS

"I don't know why I'm not healing! SIBO and candida keep coming back, no matter how clean I eat or the supplements I take." Jess, a new client, told me in our first session. I was not the first person she had come to for help, but I was determined to be the last. Everything about the way she delivered this message gave me a good indication as to one of the root causes behind her problem.

"Jess, I hear you. I am so sorry this is your experience. I really do think we need to talk about stress. Stress plays such a huge role in our healing."

"I hear you, But I'm not stressed—at least no more than the average person." Then, she paused. "Okay... I'm stressed over this if anything!"

"Stress is really tricky. We can *think* we aren't stressed but still be sending signals to our body that we are. Thing is, your brain can't tell the difference between running from a bear versus '*Should I eat that sweet potato or not?*'

"I'd like you to try this experiment. I'm going to time you for one minute. Count your number of breaths for me."

After a minute, she counted 48 breaths. This was the eye-opener that allowed her to visually see her stress. This is because the ideal breath rate at rest is four to seven breaths per minute. This rate signals "Hakuna Matata" to the body.

Jessica was running from a bear on the inside. This is the message that she was giving her body with such a rapid rate of breathing. Remember, stress stinks for your microbiome.

## BREATH: THE BEST THING BEFORE SLICED BREAD.

We can go three weeks without food and sleep and three days without water, but we can only go a few minutes without breathing and the oxygen that air contains.

Your breath, specifically oxygen, is the *most* powerful tool that you possess to spark gut healing, manage stress, and calm a hyperactive HPA axis (your stress response system). There's a reason that athletes will spend hours in an oxygen tent to overcome an injury in time for the big game.

Each time you inhale air, you take in the oxygen that your body needs to function. The more your body is in "repair" mode, the more oxygen you need, and the more efficiently you can deliver oxygen to your muscles, the better and more efficiently your body can repair, ultimately leading to better health restoration.

A lack of oxygen due to chronic inflammation and stress increases inflammatory cytokines in the body and plays an important role in disease pathogenesis. Interestingly, many gram-negative gut bacteria and parasites are anaerobic in nature, meaning they thrive upon a *lack* of oxygen. This is perhaps why patients with IBD (including Crohn's and colitis) experience decreased inflammation and remission of flares with hyperbaric oxygen therapy, a modality originally designed for individuals recovering from traumatic brain injuries. Hyperbaric-oxygen-treated colitis patients showed 63 percent better recovery rates during flares, compared to only 10 percent of IBD patients using traditional steroid therapy.

When we uptake pure oxygen and breathe more deeply, oxygen enters the tissues of the body where it attacks and kills bacterial and yeast overgrowth, fungus, mold, and toxic pathogens—all with an intense and short-lived die-off and without negative effects on the liver. Hence, *increased* oxygen delivery to the tissue may reverse the pathological process. Oxygen supports the immune system, neutralizes toxic substances, fuels metabolism, and promotes new cell growth. Oxygen also stimulates the creation of new blood vessels and red blood cells to carry oxygen throughout the body for repair, including repair to your gut lining.

Fitness enthusiasts with increased VO2 maxes—maximal oxygen uptake which is connected to better endurance and overall fitness—*also* have healthier, balanced gut microbiomes. In a study of 37 healthy male and female gym warriors, researchers found that those with better aerobic endurance (oxygen uptake) during training *also* had a greater abundance of healthy bacteria in their gut. Moreover, there was *no* correlation between body weight, macronutrients, or body fat and better gut microbiomes in the athletes, meaning that just because one person looks lean, eats fewer carbs, or has more muscle, it doesn't necessarily mean they are fitter or have a healthier gut (but if they have better quality oxygen uptake, they may).

Breathing is something you do more than *twenty thousand* times per day. So, how are you breathing?

The quality of your breathing in your daily life can get you better results with your Total Gut Reset.

## BREATHING PROPERLY.

Although it may sound crazy to think that there's a right and wrong way to breathe, there is.

Common signs of improper breathing include:

- Inhaling with your chest;
- Mouth breathing;
- Rapid short breaths;
- Tight shoulders and upper neck muscles;

- Slouching;
- Frequent yawning;
- A high resting breath rate (over 12 breaths per minute);
- A non-expanding rib cage when you breathe.

On the other hand, proper breathing looks like sitting up straight and diaphragmatic breathing, not chest breathing or breathing that involves shoulder movement. If you fully expand your rib cage by taking a deep breath, you should see your belly rise. Inhale through the nose and exhale through the nose or mouth. Ideally, inhale for five to ten seconds and exhale for the same length of time. Aim for no more than five to seven breaths per minute during rest or normal daily activities in order to achieve the parasympathetic state. This state signals "calm" to your body.

As for exercise and activity, the number one goal is no panting when exerting yourself. Breathe deeply and calmly from the diaphragm, not your chest, by inhaling through your nose when you can and exhaling upon exertion. In general, the rib cage should expand in a 3D pattern, from top to bottom, back to front, and to the sides. Control your breath by consciously cuing yourself to make each breath you take in equal to each breath you push out, and try not to hold your breath as much as possible.

If you struggle to take deep breaths in through your nose, try nasal breathing strips like "Breathe Right" at night time to open up air pathways.

## AIR QUALITY MATTERS

Beyond our personal breathing abilities, the quality of the air we breathe also matters—especially our *indoor* air quality.

While outdoor air pollution and seasonal allergens, like pollen and outdoor molds, matter too, most people spend up to 22 hours a day, or over 90 percent of their time, indoors where molds, mycotoxins, gas emissions, electromagnetic fields, and other air pollutants can prompt inflammation and weaken detoxification pathways.

The concentrations of these air pollutants may be two-and-a-half times higher indoors than outdoors and trigger the onset of gut disorders by altering immune gene expression, spiking inflammation, and increasing gut permeability. Additionally, it's been estimated that more than 50 percent of all buildings in the US have water damage and mold and that more than 10 million people suffer from mold illness due to long-term exposure.

Mold and mycotoxicity are often the elephants in the room that most doctors, even holistic doctors, are not looking for when a patient presents with gastrointestinal distress and a host of other symptoms.

The main reason mold is detrimental is the toxic mold spore by-products, known as mycotoxins. Mycotoxins are toxic to humans and are best known for their uses in manufacturing chemical and biological warfare weapons. Unfortunately, mycotoxins are tiny, as small as 0.1 microns, making them invisible to the naked eye. For context, their big brother, a grain of sand, is sixty microns, and a single human hair is about one hundred microns thick. Mycotoxins are also heavy, meaning they easily fall to the ground and take up residence wherever they land, particularly thriving on porous items such as clothing, furniture, wood, upholstery, carpet, and paper. This is the opposite of the many allergens and pollutants that circulate in the air and are more easily filtered with a good HEPA filtration system and an air purifier.

Studies show that after just one week of exposure to ochratoxin–a mycotoxin commonly found in millions of homes nationwide and often in foods like coffee, oats, corn, wheat, nuts, and beans–healthy bacteria *permanently* disappeared, accompanied by a significant reduction in total short-chain fatty acids that guard against toxins. In another report on exposure to the mycotoxin trichothecenes–a derivative from black mold–researchers noted a two- to three-fold rise in bacteria synonymous with SIBO, as well as leaky gut and increased cortisol (inflammation) throughout the body.

High amounts of electromagnetic field (EMF) exposure also creates oxidative stress for our gut biome.

EMFs come from cell phones, cell towers, Wi-fi, and 5G networks, and although they are around most of us all the time, researchers speculate that one day EMFs will be called the "cigarettes of the 1950s".

Your body responds to EMFs because, being 70 percent water, it is an excellent conductor of electricity. Man-made EMFs change the natural electrical currents in our bodies, altering the function of our cells and organs. Common symptoms reported with frequent or compounded EMF exposure include tingling, muscle twitching, headaches, poor sleep, hormone imbalances, and digestion difficulties (IBS, diarrhea, constipation). EMFs inhibit the growth of beneficial gut bacteria, trigger dysbiosis, and increase antibiotic resistance.

Now imagine someone who carries their mobile phone in their pocket every day or someone who sits with their laptop on their lap while it is connected to the Wi-fi. In a study on bacteria and its response to 5G radiation, researchers noted a significant increase in the growth of glucose-hungry microbes and yeast after just eight hours of exposure—two-thirds the average time spent on a screen during the day.

Although mold and EMFs are not going anywhere soon, the more distance you keep from them, the better. Keep your air squeaky clean and keep your phone away from your body (for example, out of your pockets). Use speakerphone in lieu of Bluetooth. Also, keep your phone and devices out of your bedroom and disconnect your Wi-Fi at night to avoid unnecessary voltage and EMFs.

## BREATHING (IN YOUR MIND) MATTERS TOO

Perceived psychological stress has a huge impact on Secretory IgA levels (sIgA)—a marker of gut inflammation. One study took a group of teens, put them in a room, and had them watch nothing but acts of violence on TV for two hours. Researchers then measured their sIgA levels that day and the next day, and they dropped—low sIgA indicates *increased* inflammation. After that, the researchers put them in a room again, and they only watched happy, peaceful acts of human kindness on TV, and their sIgA levels went up, indicating decreased inflammation.

Another study in fifty IBS and IBD patients found that the participants who participated in an eight-week mindfulness training (compared to non-mindfulness-trained patients) experienced a significant decrease in fecal calprotectin and C-reactive protein—markers typically associated with excess bloating, diarrhea, and constipation. Even six months later, these changes remained without any other change in diet, medication, or exercise.

## TRANSLATION: YOUR INNER GAME AFFECTS YOUR INNER GUT GAME.

Thanks to the Gut-Brain Connection—our minds have *amazing* control over our physical bodies. Your body is objective. It doesn't know the difference between an actual experience in your life that creates an emotion and an emotion you've created by thought alone. Our bodies cannot differentiate between physical factors that make us stressed—such as under-sleeping, overtraining, and standing outside in blistering heat versus the anxious thoughts that create stress. To our bodies, the feeling is just *stress*—no matter what it took to get to that point. So, to convince our bodies to feel at ease, we are required to use conscious effort to shift from a primitive response to a parasympathetic nervous system response, in which you rest and digest.

A simple way to "just breathe in your mind" is by adopting the concept of *cause vs. effect*. Are you happening to the day, or is the day happening to you?

A Cause vs. Effect mindset is all about how you see daily life and situations. Is the glass half full or half empty? How can you proactively generate more positive, favorable outcomes, even when life doesn't go as planned?

For example, two people can be sitting in rush hour traffic, both running behind to their next appointment, and have a completely different experience.

The person in **Effect** has a meltdown—*Why* is this happening TO ME?! They wonder as they flip off the guy who blinks in front of them and honk at the person in front of them while traffic is at a standstill. Clearly, the world is not on their side.

The person at **Cause**, on the other hand, is equally running late; however, they put on their "at cause" mindset and think a few things:

- There's nothing I can do about this traffic. I am thankful I will at least get there safely;
- Just breathe;
- What can I do with this time? (Maybe listen to a podcast or catch up with a good friend on the phone).

A **Cause** vs. **Effect** mindset can occur in any situation, and we get an insurmountable number of daily opportunities to practice it.

For example, a friend has a repeated habit of not texting you back. An **Effect** mindset would convince you that she must be mad at you. Or, it may lead you to ask, "What did I do wrong?" A **Cause** mindset, however, would encourage you to think differently: She must be busy or have a lot going on in her life; I choose to surround myself with people in my inner circle who are reciprocal.

Another example: Your weight loss efforts aren't working. An **Effect** mindset would tell you that when life slows down, I can focus (everything is always getting in my way). A **Cause** mindset is: What is one small step I can take today toward my goals? Or, what are my personal roadblocks that I repeatedly run into, and how can I change one today? You can apply these principles to a myriad of other scenarios.

Although forming a new inner habit to "breathe" does not happen overnight, interjecting small "daily breath break" practices into your daily routines, such as a couple of minutes of conscious breathing, sauna sweat sessions, more laughter, meditation, breathwork or yoga, "recess breaks" to workout for fun and flow, can dramatically transform how you feel, doubling the resiliency of your gut-immune system and lowering inflammatory markers like cortisol, C-reactive protein, cholesterol, and elevated blood sugar.

Additionally, did you know that the act of simply *thinking* about something that you're grateful for boosts vagus nerve function and serotonin production—the feel-good brain chemical produced in your gut? In one study on heart failure patients, wherein half of the participants logged the things they were grateful for each day and the other half did not find that, after eight weeks, patients in the gratitude group experienced better heart health, digestion, and less anxiety overall. I keep a daily bullet journal in the notes on my phone to log at least three gratitudes for the "cool little things" that happen each day and also "brain dump" worries and prayers out of my head onto digital "paper."

And if you need some extra inspiration, 28 Olympic Medals winner in swimming Michael Phelps was well known for his pregame visualization practice during his competition years, a process involving relaxing and repeatedly programming his subconscious brain to see, smell, taste, and feel a first-place podium finish in his mind, hundreds of times before race day. By default, his body would go on autopilot to win, knowing exactly what to do as a result of repetitive mental rehearsal. Visualization allows your subconscious mind to store and remember everything you are picturing.

Ultimately, "just breathing," as both a physical and mental practice, is all about finding what works for you.

## GUT LOVE HABIT #1: JUST BREATHE

Pause to take four to seven deep breaths before each meal to put your body into "rest and digest" mode. Keep in mind that the ideal breath rate is four to seven deep breaths per minute at rest. Focus on breathing in through your nose for five to ten seconds and out through your mouth for the same amount of time.

Next Level: Take a "breath break." Establish a phone-free morning routine to get your mind and body prepped for the day ahead, such as five to ten minutes of prayer or meditation, sun salutations, or an energy-boosting workout and listening to a song or playlist that gets you pumped.

## GUT RESET EXPERIMENT: BREATH TEST

Time yourself for one minute and count the number of breaths you take in that minute. Better yet, get someone else to count them for you–you may change your pattern if you are conscious of it.

Try the following three exercises to help you retrain your breathing, so you can breathe better and more deeply at rest.

### *EXERCISE 1: 4-7-8 BREATHING:*

This is a simple cadence style of breathing you can do anytime, anywhere, to help deepen your casual breathing practice.

1. Place the tip of your tongue against the ridge of tissue behind the upper front teeth;
2. Inhale quietly through the nose and exhale audibly through the mouth;
3. Then inhale for a count of four;
4. Hold your breath for a count of seven;
5. Exhale through your mouth, making a whooshing sound for a count of eight;
6. Repeat this cycle at least three more times.

## *EXERCISE 2: BREATH WALK (OR RUN):*

Synchronize your breath with walking steps and focused attention.

## *EXERCISE 3: YOGI BREATHING:*

You don't have to take a yoga class to integrate alternate nasal breathing into your daily routine.

1. Press your thumb to your right nostril, holding it shut, and breathe out gently through your left nostril;
2. Gently inhale through your left nostril for five to ten seconds. Then, press the left nostril closed with a finger;
3. Remove your thumb from the right nostril and exhale from it for five to ten seconds;
4. Still holding your nostril shut, inhale through your right for five to ten seconds, close the nostril, and then exhale out the left for five to ten seconds;
5. Continue alternating. Continue with this pattern of alternating between nostrils for 5-10 complete rounds.

# CHAPTER 12:
# SUPERPOWER 2: HYDRATION

***"When the well's dry, we know the worth of water."***
***– Benjamin Franklin***

All life is formed in water. We would not have life without it, and there is a natural Superpower in water that most humans are unaware of—at least three in four, the same amount who are dehydrated.

One scientist, Dr. Masaru Emoto, set out to change this in the early 2000s.

Dr. Emoto was a Japanese scientist fascinated by water's power and dedicated his career to studying it. Of his most notable discoveries, which was later the subject of a documentary, Dr. Emoto found that our thoughts, feelings, words, ideas, music, and even names we call water affect the molecular structure of water and thus our physical reality. In other words, one person could think positive, loving thoughts towards water, and another person could think negative, hateful thoughts about the water, and the water's color, shape, symmetry, and molecular structure would profoundly change.

His first experiment involved putting distilled water into small jars, writing a word or short phrase on a label, and then taping that label to each jar. The jars were then left overnight on their own. Some of these words had positive associations, such as "self love," "beauty," "passion," and "happiness." Other jars had negative associations such as "evil," "hatred," or phrases such as "you disgust me." Each jar then had a small amount of water flash frozen in order to form crystals, which were then observed under a microscope. The results were astonishing; the positive words formed beautiful, symmetrical crystals that looked very similar to snowflakes, while the negative words were discolored, chaotic, and fragmented.

He decided to take the experiments a step further and wanted to see what would happen to a large amount of water over an extended period of time. His famous "Rice Experiment" involved putting the same amount of rice in three different jars and then adding the same amount of distilled water into the jars. He then closed the jars and labeled each jar with a different word. The first jar was labeled with the phrase "Thank You," the second jar with the phrase "You are an idiot," and the third jar was left with a blank label. Every day, for thirty days, he visited each jar and read aloud their corresponding label to the jar for one minute and tracked the changes in each jar over the month. By the end of the month, he had noticed that the water in the jar labeled "Thank You" had started to ferment, giving off a strong, pleasant aroma. The water in the jar labeled "You are an idiot" turned black with an unpleasant shape. The most interesting result was the last jar with the blank label that had been ignored the entire time. It turned into a nasty green-blue color as opposed to staying near its original color.

Dr. Emoto's work has us question that if water is affected by words, intentions, and energies, what about humans, who are mostly made of water? *If we transform the water and thoughts we are made of, what else is possible for our health?*

## THE POWER OF WATER

Do you ever feel thirsty or have sensations of thirst throughout the day? If so, you are definitely dehydrated.

Every function of the body is monitored and conducted by the flow of water. Your body is 60-70 percent water, so it needs water in order to sustain life.

Water ensures that adequate amounts of nutrients reach your organs, your food is digested properly, your brain thinks clearly, your metabolism is functioning adequately, your cells regenerate, and your body is able to efficiently detox and flush toxins through your lymphatic system. Water—not tea, not juice, not coffee—ensures your body is hydrated. In fact, coffee is a diuretic, meaning if you drink a lot of it, you're actually losing water and minerals, not getting them.

## WHY HYDRATION MATTERS FOR GUT HEALING.

A healthy lymphatic system is essential for any gut healing protocol, and is fueled by plenty of water. Your lymphatic system is composed of water. It is the largest circulatory system in your body—a widespread network of connective tissues and fluid surrounding every organ.

Like the Amazon River, the lymph system is your body's water channel *and* natural drainage system. Your lymph system helps deliver nutrients to tissues and organs throughout the body, and provides elimination pathways for "cellular trash" like bacteria, viruses, and toxins that pass through the intestines, skin, respiratory tract, lungs, and liver. Sweat, tears, and urine are all waste by-products of natural lymph cleansing.

*Fun fact: The lymph system drains three pounds of plaque and other toxins from the brain each year!*

Lymph nodes also boost immunity and help us fight infection by making white blood cells—the first line of defense against disease. Lymph fluids then transport white blood cells throughout the body as well as usher bad pathogens *out* of your system.

## IS YOUR LYMPH CLOGGED?

Lynnsey was a typical client I see: low energy, bloating, and SIBO. Long-term use of thyroid supplements that didn't seem to work. Dry, occasional reddening skin. Unwanted weight gain. Doing all the things: the autoimmune paleo protocol, yoga, and HIIT workouts, and sleeping eight to nine hours a night.

"I just feel so blah. I do everything to take care of myself, but nothing seems to help," she lamented.

"I know. You're not doing anything wrong at all. Sometimes we just have blind spots in our daily lives that can add up. Would you be up for keeping a three-day food log this week so I can be a fly on the wall?"

When I reviewed Lynnsey's food log, I noticed something that seemed key. I asked her how much water she drank daily. Her answer was around 40 ounces. I realized that she was dehydrated. She was not drinking enough water to flush toxins from her body. To top it off, she was also eating predominantly dry foods—bars, chips, and foods with little color. It's not that any of those things are bad, but our foods can also be hydrating and help cleanse our lymph system.

*The solution: More water!*

## CLEANSE CONUNDRUM

Cleanses involving supplements, "healthy" diet-specific foods, like paleo bars, and keto shakes, extra cardio and HIIT workouts, or not-eating-anything-at-all are really popular in the gut-healing world. However, sometimes in the midst of "cleansing," we miss a crucial step: Water.

My personal experience with first trying to "cleanse my gut" years ago is no exception. To remediate candida and SIBO, I instantly jumped on the bandwagon to get the "pathogens" out—whatever it took. This involved anti-fungal herbs, biofilm disruptors, a low-FODMAP and low-carb diet, cleanse supplements, The Medical Medium's popular *Liver Rescue*, foods that *only* fit the paleo, keto, or AIP approval; things that were supposed to help rid the body of excess fungi and bacteria.

I got worse. Way worse.

One day, while taking an herbal tincture, something went very, very wrong. I got a headache. A really bad headache. A head-crushing migraine that didn't go away for two weeks. Then I started seeing spots and flashes of light. My ears rang. The doctors worked me up for a concussion—maybe I'd hit my head and forgotten? CT scans and an MRI checked for tumors, while another doc evaluated me for a mini-stroke. Nothing.

Then, we figured it out: A neurotoxic event. The "die off" bacteria and yeasts in my body were not getting out, and there was only one place to go—my brain.

I needed to support my lymph system—my body's cleansing channels—if I wanted to cleanse appropriately. Lymphatic drainage and support are highly overlooked in the world of gut healing and body cleansing. Yet it is a basic necessity.

You can't go to the doctor and get a test for a clogged lymphatic system (unless perhaps you have lymphatic channels that are actually blocked or dysfunctional, resulting in swelling of the tissues, such as what happens after certain surgeries or as a result of traumatic injury). However, there are several signs and symptoms that can indicate your body's lymphatic channels are not working as they should, including:

- Frequent bloating;
- Constipation;
- Brain fog;
- Headaches;
- Swollen lymph glands or bodily swelling;
- Puffiness in the eyes or face;
- Water retention;
- Cellulite;
- Itchy or dry skin;
- Elevated cholesterol;
- Stiff joints (especially in the morning);
- Night sweats;
- Cold hands and feet;
- Low mood;
- Food sensitivities;
- Chronic sinus congestion;
- Worsened allergies;
- Comorbidities like gut dysbiosis, yeast overgrowth, and mold illness.

A clogged lymphatic system results from anything that prevents flow in the body. The usual suspects are pesticide-laden or artificially engineered packaged foods, antibiotics, environmental toxins, inadequate exercise, sleep deprivation, and, you guessed it, *dehydration*.

## DEHYDRATION IS COMMON (BUT NOT NORMAL).

Up to 75 percent of people are regularly dehydrated and do not realize it.

Although thirst is one of the final signs of dehydration, your body can become dehydrated well before you actually feel thirsty. Additionally, the same part of your brain—the hypothalamus—that signals "thirst" also is responsible for signaling hunger. Sometimes we get the two confused.

Beyond thirst, common signs and side effects of dehydration include:

- Decreased energy–everything moves more slowly when we lack water and electrolyte balance;

- Digestive dysfunction–constipation, bloating, indigestion, GERD, leaky gut, abdominal discomfort;
- Chronic pain–ailments such as headaches, back pain, neck pain, heartburn, rheumatoid pain, high blood pressure, high cholesterol, chest pains, allergies, and asthma are directly attributed to a water shortage;
- Depression and stress–since your brain is primarily made up of water, it needs water to continue to flourish and for your chemical properties to work correctly. With dehydration, the level of energy generation in the brain is decreased;
- "Morning sickness" or nausea–that feeling that a mother often experiences during pregnancy or nausea you may experience upon waking can actually be a signal of *thirst* and mineral imbalance (water balances sodium, potassium, calcium, and magnesium in your body).

## HOW MUCH WATER SHOULD YOU DRINK?

Just as there is no one perfect diet for all people, there is no one-size-fits-all approach to how much water you need. Intake depends on your body type (height, weight), activity levels, the climate you're in, and your intake of hydrating foods and minerals.

That said, a general rule of thumb is half your body weight in ounces as a starting point for the Average Joe engaging in the normal activities of daily living. Add in factors such as your physical activity and workouts (sweat), the heat or humidity in your climate, and your water needs increase—increasing water at least by 1-2 cups if just one of these is a factor.

## WARNING: BUT DON'T DRINK JUST ANY WATER...

Water contamination is rampant in our tap water supply. The Environmental Working Group has identified more than three hundred contaminants in public water nationwide—more than two hundred unregulated. Unfortunately, the majority of the contaminants detected in tap water testing earn a passing grade from federal and state regulatory agencies. The U.S. Environmental Protection Agency has *not* added a new contaminant to the list of regulated drinking water pollutants in more than 20 years, meaning there are no legal limits for the more than one hundred and sixty unregulated contaminants the tests detected in the nation's tap water.

Fluoride, a regulated contaminant, is another hot topic of debate. Globally, only about 5 percent of the population consumes chemically fluoridated water, with more people in the US drinking fluoride-adulterated water than all other countries combined. Once believed to help prevent mineral and bone decay, research has shown otherwise in recent years, with side effects including neurotoxicity, bone deterioration, nutrient deficiencies, thyroid dysfunction, cancer, lowered mental clarity, insulin resistance, insomnia, and heart damage. Fluoride does not undergo purification before being dumped into drinking water, as well as oral care products (that end up in our water), and it often harbors significant levels of arsenic and other heavy metal contamination.

Bottled water is not much better. Despite the marketing hype, approximately 25 percent of bottled water is sourced straight from the tap. Studies also show that bottled water samples can contain phthalates, molds, benzene, and even arsenic—a heavy metal.

## DRINK CLEAN WATER

The cleanest sources of water are filtered, purified water sources. Water filter types vary, from pitchers to containers that sit on the counter to tanks under the sink to whole house filtration systems. Filter technologies range from carbon filters to ceramic, deionization, ozone, reverse osmosis, water softeners, and more. Some remove a lot of contaminants, while others remove very little. All options have pros and cons and can be quite overwhelming if you go down the Dr. Google research rabbit hole.

So which water filter is *best*? Again, like many things health-related: there is no one-size-fits-all approach. Choosing the right water filter comes down to several considerations, including price, technology, type (countertop, pitcher, under the sink, etc.), and your lifestyle. To help you make the best choice, check out the Environmental Working Group and National Sanitation Foundation's online guides.

After conducting a ton of research and considering my on-the-go lifestyle, I came up with a few top picks, settling on a few different options for all lifestyles and budgets, including pure mineral spring water (no plastic bottles) from a reputable source (like Mountain Valley Spring or Alive Water), reverse osmosis filtration with added humic and fulvic minerals and the Berkey Water Filter—an activated carbon and fluoride-removal filter that eradicates many bacteria, fluoride, arsenic, and other heavy metal ions (as long as you clean it regularly to prevent mold growth). For in-a-pinch moments (like travel), I reach for alkaline water (if you *do* have to buy bottled water, like at the airport, opt for alkaline if they have—which helps neutralize toxins from plastics).

## ALSO, DON'T FORGET...EAT HYDRATING FOODS

Aside from water, the foods we eat also contribute to the overall water content we consume. Hydrating foods (especially veggies and fruits) contain higher water content than dry foods (such as nuts, grains, bars, shakes, meat, cheese, and packaged or processed foods) and help hydrate and flush your system.

Unfortunately, only one in ten people eat the recommended number of veggies (three to five servings per day)—even those on otherwise healthy diets. Often, when I look at the food logs of new clients who can't figure out *why* they still feel constipated, bloated, or their skin breaks out, a common theme in their daily eating habits reveals a low intake of hydrating foods in their diet—paleo crackers and cheese puffs, nut and quinoa bars, protein shakes, gluten-free pizzas, beef jerky, butter coffee, keto treats, bacon and sausage, and rice and bean bowls. Hydrating veggies, fruits, and healthy fats and fluids are lubricants for the digestive tract and lymphatic system.

# AND REMEMBER YOUR MINERALS!

Minerals are essential nutrients—like sodium, potassium, phosphorus, magnesium, sulfur, and calcium— found in food, water, and supplements that act like the "spark plugs" for the body. Minerals make things work.

Minerals are necessary to help your body "digest" and actually absorb your water in the first place, as well as maintain fluid balance (electrolytes) and a healthy pH (acidity-alkaline balance) in the body, helping prevent yeast overgrowth and bacterial infections, microbial imbalances, and nutrient deficiencies. We've all seen a TUMS or Pepto-Bismol commercial where inflammation (acidity) builds in the esophagus or stomach. Those actors do not have a healthy pH balance.

Minerals also aid your body in things you typically don't think twice about like, including:

- Maintaining a healthy heart rate and blood pressure;
- Building muscle tone;
- Firing neurons in your brain to think clearly and sharply;
- Balancing hormones, adrenals, and blood sugar;
- Keeping hair and skin healthy;
- Producing digestive enzymes, breaking down food to prevent bloating, aiding in GI motility and helping you poop.

Mineral deficiencies are epidemic in the modern day primarily due to missing minerals in our soil and food sources. We are eating and drinking but starving and dehydrating at a cellular level.

A few easy ways to optimize your mineral balance include:

- Adding a generous pinch of Himalayan pink sea salt to your morning 16 oz of lemon water and salting your food to taste;
- Eat a balanced, varied nutrient-dense diet, and aiming to eat local and/or organic as much as possible (discussed in Superpower Four);
- Add a dropper dose of humic and fulvic mineral drops to a 20 to 40 ounce water bottle to drink throughout the day
- Ditch the Gatorade for natural electrolytes. Great electrolytes options include: a pinch of sea salt, or coconut water with a pinch

of sea salt, pure celery juice, 500 to 1000 mg buffered vitamin C which contains calcium, magnesium and potassium, 200 to 300 mg drops of magnesium chloride or magnesium bath salts, and/or a homemade electrolyte drink of green or herbal tea plus humic and fulvic minerals, a splash of pineapple juice or fresh pressed orange juice, and drop of stevia to taste.

## GUT LOVE HABIT #2: HYDRATE

Aim to drink half your bodyweight in ounces of clean water daily, starting off with 16 ounces of warm lemon water first thing in the morning (before coffee).

Tip: Add a pinch of sea salt if you tend to wake up groggy and tired to balance cortisol levels.

### *GUT RESET EXPERIMENT: REPLACE COFFEE*

To revitalize your hydration status and energy levels, stick to one cup of quality organic coffee per day (be a coffee snob), or cut the coffee altogether for at least seven days.

Replace coffee *or* additional cups of coffee with more hydrating sips: water with cucumber or citrus, celery juice, ginger, and other herbal teas, and coffee substitutes like "cacao coffee," mushroom coffee, and a dandelion and chicory blend that tastes like coffee.

Coffee is not a bad thing. Too much coffee—even decaf coffee—is not a good thing.

For one, coffee is a natural gallbladder stimulator, provoking the gallbladder to produce waste and poo. So, yes, morning coffee poos are a thing! If we drink a lot of it, we can become dependent on it in order to go for a number two because we end up constipated without it. Additionally, coffee stimulates the liver to break down toxins. If you are "super-sensitive" to caffeine and lots of coffee, there's a good chance coffee is forcing your liver to break down toxins at a faster rate than you are able to clear them.

On the flip side, if you have a high coffee tolerance and "need" coffee to function for energy, you're the opposite—you don't break down toxins or stimulants well, so you need more caffeine to jumpstart the process. Coffee messes with blood sugar too. As coffee spikes cortisol, blood sugar follows suit, followed by a crash as cortisol falls down shortly after drinking it. Lastly, coffee happens to be one of the top cross-contaminated food sources with gluten and mycotoxins, especially if consumed in instant coffee form, like Folgers in your cup.

Pro Tip: Bust coffee-withdrawal headaches and coffee-withdrawal constipation.

## HACK FOR COFFEE WITHDRAWAL HEADACHES

Supplement with either a phenylalanine or a tyrosine amino acid.

Caffeine withdrawal happens in large part because the brain becomes depleted of the amino acids tyrosine and phenylalanine, leaving it unable to produce adequate amounts of dopamine. The lack of dopamine leaves you feeling sluggish, depressed, and wanting more coffee. Caffeine temporarily alleviates these symptoms by forcing the brain to produce dopamine using what little tyrosine and phenylalanine it has left—making you more dependent on coffee.

To hack this, buy a bottle of phenylalanine or tyrosine and take the five-day coffee reset challenge by replacing coffee with herbal tea, water, mushroom coffee, and/or cacao-based coffee, along with amino acid supplementation:

Day 1: 1000 mg (usually two capsules) in the morning, 1000 mg after lunch;
Day 2: 1000 mg in the morning, 500 mg after lunch;
Day 3: 500 mg in the morning, 500 mg after lunch;
Day 4: 500 mg in the morning;
Day 5: 500 mg in the morning.

## HACK FOR COFFEE WITHDRAWAL CONSTIPATION

If you're like many people, you rely on coffee to go number two. In fact, coffee makes one in three people poop shortly after consuming it.

When you drink coffee, it activates natural chemicals in your GI tract called gastrin and cholecystokinin to stimulate muscle contractions in the colon—triggering a bowel movement within 20 minutes of downing your cup of Joe. Coffee is also a bile stimulator, aiding your gallbladder to produce waste. When your gallbladder isn't producing enough bile, or it is too thick to flow freely (peanut butter vs. water-like), fat can build up in the intestinal wall and cause slower movements through the digestive tract, therefore, causing constipation and explaining why many coffee drinkers claim they can't go for a number two without coffee. Hence, if the only time you poop is *if* you drink coffee, it's a sign your gallbladder is sluggish on its own, and, more than likely, you're dehydrated.

What to do about it? Drink *plenty* of water, along with optimizing your minerals with Himalayan sea salt and supplementing with magnesium citrate, buffered vitamin C, or both for bowel tolerance. Additionally, supplemental digestive bitters can be helpful.

## BUT I'M NOT A COFFEE DRINKER!

Not a coffee drinker? Then further optimize your overall hydration and mineral status by adding in 8-16 oz. of celery juice and/or 1-2 cups of bone broth daily in addition to your water intake.

Also, take inventory of whether you're eating a hydrating or drying diet. Many people fall into the rut of eating lots of dry, hard, brown, and packaged foods without realizing those foods clog their digestive system. Take an assessment of what hydrating foods you eat each day:

- How many different colors are there?
- How many tan, brown, and white foods are you eating?
- How about packaged or processed foods (including paleo or keto nuts, bars, and shakes)?
- Are you eating a variety of essential fatty acids?

The answer for optimal hydration from food lies in color.

## THE BOTTOM LINE

Your body needs water to boost digestive enzyme production, aid in GI motility, optimize nutrient absorption, and flush toxins and pathogens out.

# CHAPTER 13:
# SUPERPOWER 3: DIGEST

No detox, medication, or diet can achieve lasting results without better digestion, as the body must be able to use the nutrients given.

You've probably heard the saying, "You are what you eat." Eat a potato chip or greasy French fries, and you'll feel like a potato chip or greasy French fries. Eat an apple or drink celery juice and feel refreshed and cleansed.

This saying isn't quite accurate, though. You aren't what you eat; you are what you *digest* and absorb. "Absorption" is a fancy word for *digestion*—the uptake and breakdown of your nutrients.

Obviously, in a book on gut health, good digestion is the name of the game. If you're not digesting your food well, then you won't obtain the maximum benefits from your nutrients, no matter how "clean" you eat. Fortunately, you have the ability to boost digestion by supporting your body's natural "digestive mechanics" with two essentials:

1. Proper food chewing and posture;
2. Stomach acid, bile, and digestive enzymes;

These two essentials are like the mechanics in your digestion factory assembly line for an optimal finished product.

## SQUATTY POTTY SUCCESS

Judy Edwards, 60, was constipated her whole life. To remedy the problem, Judy had done it all. Prune juice. Supplements. Magnesium. Fiber. No fiber. Age only made the problem worse.

Then, a doctor recommended Judy use a footstool to raise her knees while on the toilet. She tried it, and it worked. She learned we all have a kink in our colon to maintain continence. Otherwise, we would be having uncomfortable accidents wherever we go. Most problems with the colon start where that kink is. Sitting on a toilet relaxes the kink to a point, but squatting opens everything up for better evacuation.

This new revelation inspired her entrepreneurial son Bobby to begin thinking outside the box—*how can we help others poop better?*

Bobby, Judy, Judy's husband, and their other six kids began giving footstools to friends, who considered them gag gifts until they started using them. The results were effective, and the feedback they received from others was unparalleled. So Judy's family took $35,000 to set up a website and begin manufacturing. The Squatty Potty was born and quickly surged to a million-dollar product within 24 hours of appearing on the TV show *Shark Tank.*

*How* we support digestion is just as important as *what* we eat.

## DIGESTION ESSENTIAL 1: CHEW YOUR FOOD AND SIT UP STRAIGHT:

How many times do you typically chew your food?

You probably heard it a thousand times from your mom at the dinner table: "Slow down and chew your food!"

Chewing is one of the most functional aspects of our digestion, yet many of us eat quickly, hurrying through meals because of hectic schedules. When I first learned this, I became aware of how others ate. As I've already mentioned, sitting at Whole Foods Market in downtown Austin, writing this book, I couldn't help but notice CEO Tom next to me, inhaling his salad three bites at a time, or construction worker Joe destroying his black bean burger within 3 minutes, and blogger Sarah staring at her screen while demolishing her turkey club in five bites.

Try it for yourself next time you're out to eat or even over dinner tonight. Simply pay attention to how many times people chew their food—including yourself! Chances are you'll find that it's not much.

The initial breakdown of food starts in your mouth. Chewing signals the release of enzymes and stomach acid so that your stomach has an easier job. Additionally, the smaller the food particles are that you swallow, the better your stomach acid and small intestine can absorb nutrients from them. When you don't chew your food enough, some may go undigested and enter your bloodstream through small gaps that may exist between the enterocyte cells of the gut lining (leaky gut).

Ideally, you want food fully liquified in your mouth *before* you swallow it—which requires you to chew at least 20-30 times. (Hint: You don't want to recognize that chunk of chicken as a chunk of chicken in your mouth before you swallow it).

Also, check your posture! A vast majority of people have bad posture. "Sit up straight!" is a message you may remember your parents or teachers repeatedly telling you when you were a kid. While a straight spine at the table was more about good manners, it also was actually doing our gut a favor. Then, somewhere along the way, many adults lose the flexibility and strength to do so. Unlike young kids who are constantly moving in a variety of positions (sitting, crawling, walking, running, rolling, jumping, exploring, etc.), we adults are pretty stagnant. We hunch, we get "tech neck," we slouch, we strain. Poor posture and digestion *do not* go hand in hand. Slouching impairs how well our diaphragm functions—the muscle that not only helps us breathe but also supports the contractions that move food through the digestive tract.

## DIGESTION ESSENTIAL 2: STOMACH ACID, DIGESTIVE ENZYMES, AND BILE:

After you chew your food, your stomach acid, digestive enzymes, and bile help to further break down your food.

Without enough chewing and without enough stomach acid, digestive enzymes, or bile, your body is forced to digest chunks of chicken, Brussels sprouts, and strawberries, eventually leading to undigested food particles in your gut and dysfunction down the road.

Food that hasn't been digested properly results in gas, bloating, and symptoms such as reflux, GERD, and constipation. If undigested food particles stick around for too long, they ferment in the gut, breeding more bacteria than should be there, leading to dysbiosis. Gut bacteria are a good thing–overgrown or imbalanced gut bacteria are not.

## STOMACH ACID BASICS

As the name implies, stomach acid is acid found in your stomach that helps break down food during the initial stages of digestion and destroys pathogens in food before your meal finds its way through your small and large intestines for the next 12-24 hours.

When we eat, stomach acid also stimulates the release of pancreatic enzymes into the small intestine to help digest carbohydrates and activates an enzyme called pepsinogen, which then becomes pepsin, an enzyme required to digest protein. In fact, eating protein stimulates stomach acid. Protein is the most bioavailable source of zinc and B vitamins—precursors for stomach acid production. Additionally, if stomach acid levels are low, so are pepsin, digestive enzyme, and bile acid levels.

## DIGESTIVE ENZYME & BILE BASICS

Digestive enzymes are helper substances that further break down the food we eat, releasing nutrients for energy production, cell growth, and repair. If you need a visual, consider enzymes as something like Pac-Man; it chomps your food. For example, amylase in your mouth digests starch. Lactase digests lactose in dairy. Lipase breaks down fats, and protease reads down proteins but not amino acids.

Additionally, although not an enzyme, bile—a sludge-like fluid responsible for digesting fats, stimulating enzyme production, and eliminating toxins and waste—is also essential. Many people with gut-related "issues" actually have a sluggish gallbladder, congested with thick bile, like peanut butter, and it's not stimulated or strong enough to "squeeze" the bile out. As already highlighted, gallbladder congestion is a big reason why some people require coffee to go number two, but it can also be why you get bad PMS symptoms at that time of the month or feel tired on top of having low T, burp or feel bloated every time you eat, increased food and chemical sensitivities, blood sugar swings from hyper or hypoglycemia (despite eating a balanced diet), or have SIBO, chronic bloating, and/or constipation.

# WHAT CAUSES LOW STOMACH ACID, DIGESTIVE ENZYMES & BILE?

Stress and inflammation strike again!

Intestinal irritation from the usual suspects suppresses your stomach acid and enzyme production (think: processed granola bars, vitamin and mineral deficiencies in the diet, tap water, pesticides, lack of sleep, inappropriate exercise, crappy coffee, alcohol, birth control pills, plastic water bottles, and improper chewing and posture).

After all, if you're running from a bear (that is, if you're stressed), do you think your body wants to chow down on a chicken breast? Nope.

If you're eating while stressed, toxins and undigested foods drain *back* from your gut to your liver, bile thickens, and the ducts in your gallbladder and pancreas are overcrowded in digestive gridlock, unable to produce enzymes to aid in digestion. Your digestive fire weakens. Food intolerances arise. You get bloated. Constipated. Gassy. Food sits in your stomach. Your blood sugar rises or falls. You feel hangry. You get easily full. You feel brain fog. Your hormones go haywire. You need coffee to function. The cascade goes on, all because your digestive mechanics are "offline."

So, how do you tell if you are low in stomach acid, digestive enzymes, or bile? The list below will give you some idea based on your symptoms:

- Symptoms: bloating, gas, constipation, indigestion/heartburn after eating starch or carbohydrates.
  Deficiency: low pancreatic enzymes, low stomach acid (HCl);

- Symptom: constipation, stomach pain after eating proteins.
  Deficiency: low pepsin enzymes and proteolytic enzymes (protein-digesting enzymes, produced by the pancreas), low stomach acid (HCl);

- Symptoms: feeling nauseous or experiencing fish burps after you eat healthy fats, fatty fish (such as salmon or fatty foods), feeling bloated every time you eat, skin breakouts, hormone imbalances.
  Deficiency: sluggish gallbladder, low bile acid production;

# HOW TO ADDRESS STOMACH ACID, DIGESTIVE ENZYME, AND BILE DEFICIENCY

There are multiple ways to boost stomach acid, digestive enzymes, and bile naturally.

My top hack: Boost digestion with the apple cider vinegar "gut love shop," known for both stomach acid and enzyme-boosting properties. Just 1-2 tablespoons added to 4-8 ounces of water does the trick. Swig before or after meals and add a teaspoon of Manuka honey.

You can also eat enzyme-rich foods—foods naturally high in digestive enzymes themselves—to also help improve digestion. For best results, consume fruits alone 20- 30 minutes before or after a meal. Top sources include pineapple, papaya, mango, kiwi, raw honey, green-tipped yellow bananas, avocados, kefir, sauerkraut, kimchi, miso, and ginger.

As for the basics, drink 20 ounces of water *before* each meal. This encourages the production of more HCL and pancreatic enzymes. Also, season food with quality sea salt. We need adequate amounts of chloride to produce hydrochloric acid, and the best source of chloride is unrefined sea salt.

For gallbladder "love," eat cholagogue-rich foods, herbs, and spices for healthy bile. Cholagogues are foods that act as bile (waste) movers to decongest the sludge-like bile in your gallbladder and ensure full digestion. These foods, in addition to short-term enzyme supplementation *and* hydration *and minerals*, improve bile and lymphatic flow, so your gut is not congested in the long run. Top cholagogue foods include beets, cabbage, celery, garlic, horseradish, watercress, daikon radish, organic green apples, dill weed, caraway seed, ginger, artichoke, turmeric, cinnamon, fenugreek, and dandelion root—specifically fenugreek, ginger, and dandelion tea. These foods act as natural lubricants for clogged bile ducts, supporting normal bile flow. You can also try drinking olive oil and lemon juice. This combination exercises the liver and gallbladder to support healthy bile flow in the gallbladder and pancreas. Combine one tablespoon of olive oil with a generous squeeze of lemon juice in a shot glass of water, or use it as a dressing.

Experiment with a short-term low-FODMAP diet. Since carbohydrate malabsorption is common in those with GERD, heartburn, bloating, and other symptoms of low stomach acid, a short term low-FODMAP, paleo-based diet can be effective while you test and assess for the root causes of low stomach acid. Avoid snacking between meals to allow time for your body to digest foods properly.

Lastly, chew, chew, chew, and sit up! Maintain good posture throughout the day, especially around meal times, and don't lie down immediately after eating. If you must lie down, prop yourself up with pillows so your head and upper torso are raised to aid digestion.

## GUT LOVE HABIT 3: BOOST DIGESTION

Sit up and slow down to chew your food until it is fully liquefied—20-30 bites!

### *BONUS–ADD IN THE ONE-TWO PUNCH:*

Add in a little extra supplemental support into your daily routine with HCl (or apple cider vinegar "gut love shot"), digestive enzymes, and/or digestive bitters.

### *STOMACH ACID:*

Consume one tablespoon of apple cider vinegar (ACV) in water with meals to increase stomach acid.

Tip: add one teaspoon of pure maple syrup or honey to apple cider vinegar if you cannot stomach it, or take an HCl capsule or tablet* if you cannot tolerate ACV. *(*Not recommended if pregnant or taking PPI medications.)*

### *DIGESTIVE ENZYMES AND BITTERS:*

Take 1-2 digestive enzymes and/or 1-2 full droppers of digestive bitters with meals to assist in digestion.

# GUT RESET EXPERIMENT: THE STOMACH ACID AND THE DIGESTIVE ENZYMES CHALLENGE:

These two simple challenges can help determine whether you have the appropriate level of hydrochloric acid in your stomach for optimal digestion.

## *EXPERIMENT 1:* ***APPLE CIDER VINEGAR CHALLENGE.***

Take two tablespoons of apple cider vinegar straight on an empty stomach. Notice whether or not you experience a burning sensation.

1. **Yes, I experienced lots of burning!**

**What it means:** You need to heal your gastric lining, and you *may* be low in stomach acid.

**What to do:** Focus on gut lining supports for any gastric conditions with aids like mastic gum, l-glutamine, collagen, bone marrow, immunoglobulins, probiotics, and soluble fiber-based or resistant starch prebiotics (like sun fiber, modified citrus pectin, or glucomannan). Additionally, back down to using one tablespoon of apple cider vinegar in 4-8 ounces of water with meals; see how you tolerate it and if it helps you digest your meals. If it's still burning, drop apple cider vinegar altogether.

2. **No, I didn't feel any burning at all.**

**What it means:** Your stomach acid is *low*. You may also have a gut infection like *H. pylori* or SIBO if you regularly experience bloating, dissension, excessive fullness, GERD reflux-like symptoms, or abdominal pain when eating that need to be considered.

**What to do:** You may benefit from HCL (hydrochloric acid) over apple cider vinegar. Take one capsule of 500 mg of HCl on an empty stomach; note how you feel. If you feel burning after you try HCl, take 1-2 tablespoons of apple cider vinegar with meals, diluted in water.

If you don't feel burning within the first 5-10 minutes of taking one HCl, take one more capsule and see how you feel. If there is still no burning, take 1-3 capsules of HCl with meals and/or 1-2 tablespoons of apple cider vinegar in water with meals for 30-60 days, then retest how you feel going without it for 1-3 days.

3. **I felt good. A slight burning, but apple cider vinegar seems to help.**

**What it means:** You have moderate to low stomach acid and will benefit from a swig of ACV around meal times to aid digestion.

**What to do:** Add one tablespoon of apple cider vinegar to 4-8 ounces of water and swig before or after meals, as needed, for a little extra digestive "oomph."

Note: You can also do this with baking soda.

1. First thing in the morning (before eating or drinking), mix a quarter of a teaspoon of baking soda in 4 ounces of cold water;
2. Drink the baking soda solution;
3. Set a timer and see how long it takes you to burp. If you have not burped within 5 minutes, stop timing.

If your stomach is producing adequate amounts of stomach acid, you'll likely burp within 2-3 minutes. Any burping after three minutes may indicate a low acid level.

### *EXPERIMENT 2: DIGESTIVE ENZYMES CHALLENGE.*

Take 1-2 quality digestive enzyme capsules with meals for three days, and simply note how you feel. If bloating, gas, indigestion, or other ill side effects dissipate, you know you are on the right track.

## THE BOTTOM LINE

You are what you digest and absorb. If you're not digesting your food, then you won't obtain the maximum benefits from your nutrients, no matter how "clean" you eat. Boost your digestion by supporting your body's natural absorption abilities with proper food chewing, stomach acid, digestive enzymes, and digestive bitters.

# CHAPTER 14:
# SUPERPOWER 4: NUTRIENTS

When you eat, you not only feed yourself, you feed your gut bugs.

Aside from fecal microbial transplants (FMT), through which scientists switch out your gut bacteria with someone else's, diet is the number one intervention that has the most impact on the gut microbiome (yes, even more than probiotics). In fact, it only takes three days of following a particular diet to see big changes in our gut health.

Researchers comparing the gut microbiota of participants on a three-day plant-based diet and a three-day animal-based diet, consisting of the same amount of calories, concluded that *both* diets significantly altered the types of bacteria present along with their digestive abilities.

A plant-rich diet (consisting of veggies, fruits, rice, and lentils) decreased gram-negative bacteria and boosted short-chain fatty acids, which are associated with lower inflammation overall. However, this diet also would have decreased stomach acid and eventually decreased each subject's ability to tolerate animal proteins, which is associated with more inflammation, hair loss, pale skin, hormone imbalances, and slowed digestion.

On the animal-based diet (consisting of eggs, bacon, cured meats, cheese, pork, and beef), healthy bacteria kicked into high gear to metabolize amino acids better and to accelerate weight loss. However, the animal-based diet also resulted in fat malabsorption, a decrease in short-chain fatty acids, and an increase in gram-negative bacteria connected to intestinal inflammation, watery stools, and inflammatory bowel disease. All this after just three days of not eating fiber!

Researchers concluded that our gut bacteria change rapidly depending on the diet we feed them.

## THE TURKEY BURGER

One of my favorite foods is a turkey burger. However, during my dieting days, I took it a little to the extreme. For three years straight, I lived on turkey patties topped with rubbery fat-free Kraft cheese for breakfast, lunch, and dinner, along with Crystal Light, steamed vegetables, and artificially-sweetened whey protein powder. That's it.

And not just any turkey patty. ONLY a turkey patty from The Gym Cafe in my hometown, Little Rock, Arkansas, would do. When I went away to college and grad school, I'd pay my mom to ship out my beloved turkey patties in bulk orders of 60-90 at a time, and I stored them for months in the freezer.

The result? A famine in my gut microbiome, along with digestive distress and a host of diagnoses down the line.

*Lightbulb: Our gut bugs eat what we feed them. Long-term restrictive diets kill off many, many species and varieties of bugs in your gut.*

## HOW TO EAT FOR A HEALTHY GUT

"I am so confused about what to eat," said *you* (and most people)!

According to a survey by the Food International Council Foundation, 80 percent of all Americans report being utterly confused about what being healthy even means due to conflicting health information. Only about one in three people can identify even one food that would be best for their body and their unique health goals.

There are *hundreds* of different philosophies, protocols, and prescriptions out there claiming to be "The Way." However, if no two humans are alike, what makes us believe that one dietary approach is the panacea for a particular goal or condition?

*This is the main reason why diets fail—even supposed "gut healing" diets.*

The term "diet failure" doesn't just refer to throwing in the towel. I've had clients who maintained restrictive low histamine, low FODMAP, anti-candida, specific carbohydrate diet, keto approach, AIP protocol, or other diets for years and completely adapted to eating a limited food selection, but their gut microbiome still was *not* better. Not healed. They may have felt better at first—during the initial 3-6 months—but as the limited diet became their new norm, some gut and health symptoms remained. Other new symptoms arose.

*This is exactly what happened to me.*

In my recovery from my extreme dieting days and eating disorders, as I transitioned from the extreme Pop-Tart and Egg McMuffin diets my dietician prescribed me in treatment, I instantly felt better. Eating real food really does a body—and gut biome—good!

However, as time went on, to further improve the autoimmune diseases I developed during my treatment, I transitioned to an autoimmune paleo diet. Again, I instantly felt better, at least initially.

Little did I realize that the AIP approach further reduced the diversity of my gut microbiome the longer I followed the diet. Instead of focusing on addressing and healing my gut health with additional supports, like probiotics, boosting stomach acid and enzyme production, liver and lymph cleansing support, and gut lining restoration, I relied on the restrictive diet to fix me. In the long run, I became intolerant to more and more foods. Oxalates in spinach gave me IBS. Fermented foods gave me asthma. Red meat sat in my stomach, feeling like a brick. Macadamia nuts made me itch. The whole purpose of the elimination diet missed the mark entirely.

A good sign of a "healthy" gut is a gut that tolerates *more*, not fewer, nutrients—even the occasional burger and sweet potato fries out at your favorite local Burger Up restaurant, a scoop of real ice cream, or movie-theater-worthy homemade popcorn with real butter or coconut oil; an 80/20 balance. Sure, you may feel "off" when you eat "off," but if your gut is not "wrecked" by the occasional "not-right-now" food, this is the metabolic flexibility of a resilient gut.

Unfortunately, our culture has strayed away from the original meaning of the word "diet," which stems from the Latin *dieta*. This translates to "way of life." Long before Whole30 rule books or conflicting low histamine and anti-candida protocols floated around on the interwebs, humans ate a variety of nutrient-dense whole foods with one ingredient in season and did not discriminate or judge food based on the latest fad diet claim.

Ultimately, to establish a nutritional baseline for your gut bugs, practice one principle: Eat whole, nutrient-dense foods with the least-restrictive mindset possible. Focusing on whole, nutrient-dense foods cuts out the gray zone of wondering whether a daily handful (or bag full) of Goldfish crackers with a twenty-year shelf life is really a way of life.

In practice, the best way I have found to do this entails knowing exactly how your gut bugs operate and how to use food to cultivate a healthy gut.

## CULTIVATING A HEALTHY GUT WITH FOOD: SEVEN UNIVERSAL TRUTHS

The nutrients in our diet are like using nutrient-dense soil, sunlight, and mineral-rich water to grow a beautiful garden.

What happens to your flowers if you dump gasoline on them? They die. What happens if you leave your flowers in the dark? They wilt. What happens if you don't water or feed your plants at all?

Likewise for your gut biome.

You have trillions of "buddies in your belly"—gut bugs. What would it be like to think about feeding them when you feed yourself? To do this effectively, it's important to know what these little critters like to eat. Although nutrition research is ongoing, several universal truths apply to happy gut bugs.

### *TRUTH 1: GUT BUGS REQUIRE FOOD DIVERSITY*

Variety and diversity are the spice of life. Of the trillions of bacteria in our gut, you can bet that not every single one doesn't thrive from eating chicken and broccoli every single day. Imagine if you ate the same chicken and broccoli for three meals a day, every day. You would grow bored and sick of that meal. A thriving gut microbiome needs variety, too. Studies in women with anorexia—known for restrictive diets consisting of only 5-10 foods—reveal significant dysbiosis and low bacterial diversity when compared to subjects who are of normal weight, obese, or athletes.

There is no shortage of gut-nourishing foods on the planet; however, the average American isn't consuming them.

- Of the three hundred thousand known edible plant species, humans only use two hundred;
- Six livestock breeds are lost each month in favor of high-production practices;
- Seventy-five percent of the world's food is generated from only twelve plants and five animal species.

What about restrictive and elimination diets? Those are used all the time for therapeutic dietary protocols. The low FODMAP diet, for example, may help silence symptoms of bloating and constipation. However, it may have long-lasting consequences due to negative long-term shifts in the gut microbiome.

How to safely use an elimination diet:

- Take a short-term approach with it;
- Simultaneously address underlying causes of gut imbalance;
- Follow with a reintroduction of whole, nutrient-dense foods.

## *TRUTH 2: GUT BUGS NEED THE REAL THING*

There's a difference between an apple and an apple pie. You know this, and so do your gut bugs. The same goes for enriched-wheat snack crackers and five-ingredient, seed-based crackers sold at your local health food store. The more whole and less processed, the better. Ideally, choose foods that contain five ingredients or less, or have no label at all.

## *TRUTH 3: GUT BUGS REALLY LOVE FIBER*

Contrary to popular no-carb and low-carb diet hype, if there is *one* food that is associated with an increase in microbial diversity and healthy bacteria (along with a host of other side effects such as reduced inflammation, weight loss, and improved immune function and digestion) it is carbs—specifically prebiotic fibers and carbohydrates that foster the growth of short-chain fatty acids.

Carbohydrates are the principal energy source for forming healthy microbes, and prebiotic fibers are arguably more important than probiotics (since they help your probiotics stick in the first place). PubMed boasts over four thousand studies alone on the topic. And today, while the most consumed foods in the American diet include pizza, bread, high-fructose corn syrup (sweetener), grain-based desserts, alcohol, orange and apple juice (for our fruits), and potatoes and tomatoes (for veggies), the top foods of our healthy ancestors were based on a primarily plant-based diet (starchy plants, leaves, nuts and seeds, fruits). The average ancestral diet included 100 grams or more of fiber a day. The average American diet includes only 8-15 grams of fiber.

*Dilemma: "But I feel worse when I eat carbs (including fiber rich veggies)!"*

This is a common phenomenon that many with gut issues experience, especially those with gut infections, small intestinal bacterial overgrowth, blood sugar imbalances, dysbiosis, or other gut pathologies. The key here is not that carbs are innately bad, but instead that they may not be good for you right now, at least until you address the underlying imbalance.

## TRUTH 4: GUT BUGS GET CONFUSED EASILY

Feed your bugs chocolate ice cream every night after dinner, and what do you think your gut bugs are going to want to eat every night after dinner? Chocolate ice cream.

Our cravings and the types of foods we like to eat are a direct by-product of the soil "tilling" we do day in and day out in the food choices we make. Considering that the foods we eat alter the types of gut bacteria living inside us, it makes sense then that our biome's species adapt to whatever you feed them over time.

Ever known a kid who said, "I don't like broccoli?" Kids and adults with strong aversions to foods like broccoli or Brussels sprouts are called Supertasters because, as we have discussed, they have higher amounts of certain bacteria dictating their food preferences. Their gut bugs give them lower thresholds for tolerating sweet, sour, salty, and bitter tastes than non-Supertasters.

## TRUTH 5: GUT BUGS RUN ON A SCHEDULE

Your bodily processes run according to a circadian rhythm which regulates your body's energy expenditure, appetite, and sleep. Similarly, your gut bugs function according to a microbial clock—with a preference for eating, digesting, waking, sleeping, and repairing. Gut microbiota "rhythms" are expressed through the secretion of molecules at specific times of the day. For instance, at night, gut bacteria related to DNA repair, energy metabolism, and cell growth are enacted. This is why night fasting—sleeping through the night and not eating for 8-14 hours—is beneficial for the gut microbiota. It's when our bacteria produce short-chain fatty acids like butyrate, which regulates glucose levels through various glucose-related hormones, which in turn regulate fat metabolism in the liver.

Depending on how much and how well we sleep, our gut bacteria's daytime clock, metabolism, and digestion are also affected. Sleep time controls when our gut bugs like to eat, as well as when they like to eat and our blood glucose levels. Any long disruption to this cycle may contribute to an unbalanced gut microbiota, which may lead to side effects such as blood sugar imbalances, suppressed fullness cues, increased appetite, caffeine dependence, and cravings for certain foods outside of your normal diet.

Gut bugs thrive upon staying in sync with the rhythms of the sun. Digestive "fire" (efficiency of your food processing) is typically higher in the earlier part of the day—just like your energy levels—and slowly decreases in the evening hours.

What about intermittent fasting (IF), you may ask. IF is a hot topic in the microbiome world. Just as an athlete gets stronger and faster when he takes a recovery day or two off from training, IF theoretically works the same way for your gut—it gives your digestive system a break, for 12-16 hours, from constantly working out to clear out unwanted debris, excess nitrogen, reactive oxygen species, and other inflammatory proteins.

That said, the studies showing whether or not IF actually increases microbial diversity are mixed. Although some mice studies yield promising results, very few human studies have been conducted on the subject. The research we do have shows that time-restricted feeding is really only beneficial in the short-term for people who are overweight, obese, and/or have significant insulin dysregulation (although even at that, studies also suggest that results are similar to any other reduced caloric intake diet, and lost water weight may play a role).

As for the gut, IF does not significantly alter the diversity or overall composition of the microbiome long term. Just like people who eat McDonald's or chicken and broccoli every day have a different microbiome, so do intermittent fasters. However, if you change your diet, your gut shifts again. In other words: You can shape your gut with food without necessarily having to fast.

The "Goldilocks" approach is imperative with IF. Not eating or accidental dieting can have the opposite effect on microbial diversity, dampening it since gut microbes require food and fiber to survive and thrive. The best way to start IF is to simply fast overnight for 12-14 hours between your dinner, say at 8 p.m., to your morning meal at 9am the next day. Longer than that is really not necessary and may even lead to decreased energy, decreased metabolism (by 200-500 calories per day), increased social isolation, and reduced cognitive function (to think about things outside of food).

One caveat here would be if you have significant intestinal inflammation or autoimmunity of the gut—such as IBD—wherein your digestive system is begging for relief from overwork and irritation. Supervised or well-planned, short-term, and calorically adequate fasting via liquids and IF with easy-to-digest foods, like broths, stewed, slow-cooked meats, flaky fish, ghee and olive oil, and well-cooked soluble fibers, may be advised.

## *TRUTH 6: GUT BUGS DIGEST CERTAIN FOODS BETTER THAN OTHERS*

A varied diet is king in a gut-healthy diet, but not all foods digest well or digest well together. Improper food digestion can cause gas, indigestion, bloating, metabolic imbalances, and eventually speed up the process of aging. Optimize digestion by practicing some of these healthy food preparation and eating practices:

- Eat protein, healthy fat, and fiber (i.e., cooked veggies, resistant starch, fruit in a smoothie, etc.) with each meal. Simple meals digest best;
- Complex starches and proteins are best eaten in smaller amounts of each when together (i.e., a large, half-a-pound T-bone steak and football-sized sweet potato will compete with each other to digest; go for half the sweet potato or vice versa);
- Eat fruit alone earlier in the morning, as a dessert after a meal or with simple easy-to-digest foods, like tossed into a smoothie, yogurt or with a handful of nuts. Stick to 1-2 servings of fruit per day;
- Slow cook, bake, pan saute, stew, or broil meats. Avoid charred, burned, chargrilled, or overcooked meats;
- Pair protein with non-starchy veggies. Leafy greens, non-starchy vegetables, and herbs and spices go with everything;
- Cooked veggies digest better than raw. Steamed, sauteed, and slow-cooked veggies digest best;
- Eat a condiment-sized serving of fermented or pickled foods and/or apple cider vinegar "shot" with at least one meal daily;

- Add sea salt to meals to not only taste but also to absorb nutrients better;
- Drink plenty of water away from meals.

## *TRUTH 7:* ***GUT BUGS REGULATE YOUR BLOOD SUGAR AND CRAVINGS***

Your gut bacteria are the operators of your blood sugar balance and cravings. Healthy gut bacteria help keep your bacteria balanced by absorbing nutrients and appropriately using sugar energy from food.

Blood sugar is simply the concentration of glucose (sugar from food) in the blood. It is a sign of how well your body is using and digesting the nutrients you eat. Although sugar tends to get a bad rep, most foods we consume are converted into glucose (the energy we derive from food). Blood sugar is a representation of how much energy we have in our bodies at one time. Unhealthy or imbalanced gut bacteria are not able to absorb or harvest your nutrients appropriately, leading to "dysglycemia" symptoms—high or low blood sugar—like feeling shaky, lightheaded, hangry if meals are delayed, poor appetite in the morning followed by hunger at night, insomnia, hair loss, headaches, brain fog, fatigue, and cravings.

Specific types of gut bacteria send signals to your brain, telling you what they want to eat so they can boost serotonin and dopamine—the feel-good brain chemicals produced in your gut.

Studies in gastric-bypass patients and pregnant women offer great insights into the gut-cravings connection. The gut undergoes a monumental shift after bypass surgery. As a result, people suddenly stop craving Wendy's double bacon cheeseburgers and hiding Jolly Ranchers in their pockets... willpower? Or a gut shift?

Pregnancy also creates major changes in a mom's gut. Vaginal microbes transform into tons of lactobacillus species that mimic the microbiome of an obese person as their body begins to nourish another human. These gut bacteria often crave funky things like pickles and ice cream, pimento cheese sandwiches, and mac and cheese.

Another example: Do you like to eat the same foods every day? A non-diverse gut biome thrives upon a low-diverse diet, so people who tend to eat the same foods every day have less gut diversity.

What about cravings for foods that don't always make you feel great, but for some reason, you still crave them anyways, like cheese? Despite the bloating and brain fog, you can't help it because of the casomorphins—drug-like chemicals that imbalanced microbes want more of.

Gut bacteria can also dictate the foods you dislike. For example, "Supertasters" have a completely different gut bacteria profile that tells them *not* to eat bitter foods like Brussels sprouts and broccoli. A challenge I often give my patients is to make a list of the veggies they don't love and nutrient-rich foods they don't eat much of and eat more of them to diversify their gut.

The bottom line: your gut bacteria dictate your cravings, hunger cues, and energy levels by affecting your blood sugar levels, and like most gut-axis connections, imbalanced blood sugar can also cause an imbalanced gut. This is because blood sugar levels go up when cortisol goes up, causing inflammation, and we all know what excess cortisol and inflammation do to the gut via the Gut-Brain Connection.

Hence, we can inadvertently balance gut bacteria by balancing blood sugar.

## *TRUTH 8:* ***GUT BUGS ARE OMNIVORES***

From the time of your birth, you required three main nutrients to grow and function: fat, fiber (carbs), and protein. These are all found in the *perfect* human food, your mother's breast milk, consisting of about 10-20 percent protein, 50 percent fat, and 25-40% carbohydrates.

Although carbs, meats, and fats all get a bad rep depending on whether you ask a vegan, carnivore, or keto adherent, humans are omnivores. Sure, you can get carbohydrates from a chicken breast as your body converts protein into glucose, but is it ideal? Nope.

Of course, you can consume some fat—0.5 grams—in an apple, but is it a preferred source of fat? Nope.

And yes, your body can use some protein found in beans and nuts for its amino acid supply, but is it the purest source of protein? Nope, these are utilized better as fiber and fats.

Rest assured: We're not going to get into a philosophical debate on gut-healing diets or over which diet is best for you. Remember, there is no one-size-fits-all approach to the optimal human diet. However, the first universal truth hardwired into the workings of your gut biome is this: Each macro-nutrient—proteins, fats, and the fibers found in carbs—plays a unique role in cultivating a happy, healthy belly. Oh, yes, *and* probiotics.

# PROTEIN

Contrary to the popular belief that protein or meat is bad for gut health, our gut bacteria possess a very strong ability to digest and benefit from proteins. Complete proteins, found in animal products such as fish, meat, poultry, and eggs, in particular, are the major source of nitrogen for healthy colonic microbial growth—essential for the breakdown of prebiotics and plant-based carbohydrates in the first place, and also the production of beneficial short-chain fatty acids in the colon, which reduce inflammation and toxicity in the gut.

Protein is also essential for liver health and daily detoxification. A big mistake people often make when detoxing or cleansing is cutting back on protein in favor of juices, teas, and a plant-based diet. However, a protein-deficient diet impairs detox pathways in the liver and is the reason a juice fast might actually leave you worse off. You cannot effectively remove toxins without amino acids that bind the transformed toxins in the liver so they can be carried out of the body.

A review evaluating eight different high-protein diet interventions and their effect on gut bacteria composition found that higher protein diets actually have very few negative effects on gut bacteria, meaning high-protein *diets* don't diminish or cause unhealthy gut bacteria. Instead, the researchers found that different types of gut bacteria simply evolve to digest proteins, increasing certain strains while decreasing others. As long as we are eating a *balanced* diet, including carbs and fats, there is no dysbiosis created.

That said, higher protein diets (30 percent or more of your total daily caloric intake) in the absence of fiber have been correlated with increased inflammation, like IBS and IBD, which is perhaps why marketing campaigns for "Impossible Burger" claim meat is "bad" for you. Also, keep in mind that the *types* of protein you consume make a difference. Proteins containing pollutants negatively alter the gut microbiota, whereas organic pastured and wild-caught sources reduce toxic burden and microbial disruption.

## FATTY ACIDS

Quality essential fatty acids found in foods such as avocados, salmon, olive oil, coconut oil, and ghee not only act like "nutrient glue" in the digestive tract for better absorption of vitamins and minerals but also lower inflammatory markers and improve insulin (blood sugar) balance, aiding in a balanced gut ecosphere when consumed in moderate amounts.

When we eat fat, we stimulate the release of bile by the gallbladder. Low-fat diets are correlated with sluggish digestion, increased intestinal inflammation, and nutrient deficiencies primarily because optimal bile release is not triggered. Additionally, poor liver or gallbladder function also decreases bile production. In the absence of bile, fats become indigestible and are instead excreted in your poo. If you've ever had greasy, dark, foul-smelling, or clay-colored stools, poor bile production, clogged bile ducts, or fat indigestion, it's likely your liver and gallbladder are speaking.

In recent years, high-fat diets have made a comeback, boasting results such as smaller waists, coffee-less energy, and enhanced memory and libido. However, like proteins and carbs, it's important to remember that your gut thrives upon balance overall—not too much, not too little of anything for optimal gut health. Despite the hype that carbs are the enemy and fat is the fast track to dropping four dress sizes, the longer-term effects of low-carb diets on the gut are not as promising.

After six months of a high-fat diet (40 percent fats), one study showed people experienced increased leaky gut as well as increased blood sugar imbalances and insulin resistance (diabetes). For context, a keto diet is 60-70 percent fat—almost twice the fat of a non-keto diet.

Does the fat quality matter? Yes. Studies comparing a Western-based high-fat diet (rich in the saturated fats contained in hydrogenated and soybean oils) to a more well-rounded keto-paleo-style diet (a blend of saturated, monounsaturated, polyunsaturated, and omega-3 fats) show key differences in inflammatory markers (34). Additionally, the state of your gut *before* adopting a keto-based or low-carb diet matters too. This is why people typically see results within the first few months of adopting a ketogenic diet; it re-shifts their biomes in the short term before hitting a wall where weight loss, energy, metabolism, and/or digestion eventually decrease. What was once productive becomes counterproductive.

The main takeaway: Fat is the key link for nutrient synergy, specifically aiding in the absorption and uptake of vitamins and minerals.

# CARBS AND PREBIOTICS

Carbs get a bad rep. However, not all carbs are the same. Your body responds to different types of carbs in different ways—namely, *cellular* carbs and *acellular* carbs.

Traditional ancestral foods are primarily cellular carbs (roots, tubers, leaves, and fruits)—foods that contain their carbs packaged inside of cells. These cells have fiber that remains intact during cooking, decreasing the total number of carbs your body actually gets from them. Here, carbohydrate density is low. Foods with low carb density stabilize blood sugar and aid digestion, providing bulk to the stool and feeding your gut bacteria.

Acellular carbs, on the other hand, represent the majority of carbs found in modern Western diets, such as refined flour, sugar, and processed grains. These carbs don't have cell walls or have had them removed due to processing. Their high carbohydrate density contributes to elevated blood sugar and digestion difficulties. Cellular carbs help release leptin, the fullness hormone, and prevent overeating, whereas dense acellular carbs interfere with our leptin signals, resulting in the loss of fullness cues.

If all carbs led to weight gain and diseases, many indigenous populations would have a high death rate. Consider the Okinawans of Japan and the Kitavans from Papua New Guinea, who consume 65-70 percent of their energy from carbs, yet they still have a lean body mass and a low rate of disease. The key factor for keeping lean on a high-carb diet? A balanced, diverse gut microbiome.

One of the biggest differences between ancestral and current diets is how many carbs—especially fermentable fiber (prebiotics) and whole food starch—people consume. Analysis of both ancestral and modern-day hunter-gatherer diets suggests that dietary intake of inulin alone—a starchy substance found in a wide variety of fruits, vegetables, and herbs—was about 100-135 grams per day for the typical forager. Compare this with the average daily fiber intake of 10-15 grams per day in the US, and it's clear that we are a far cry from the ideal human microbiome diet.

Enter: Prebiotics and colonic foods—two sources of dietary fiber that are the biggest game changers for cultivating the *ideal* diverse human microbiome.

Prebiotics, also known as MACs (microbiota-accessible carbohydrates), are fiber-rich foods found primarily in veggies, fruits, legumes, nuts and seeds, herbs, and some properly prepared grains. Prebiotics are "selectively fermentable," meaning they feed specific types of healthy gut bacteria.

Prebiotics are *not* digested until they reach the colon, where they increase bowel mass and promote the growth of certain bacterial species. Prebiotics act like the glue that helps your probiotics stick in your gut and, by default, end up helping us digest and absorb nutrients better thanks to increased beneficial species. Prebiotic fiber also provides bulk to create picture-perfect golden stools and stimulate bile acid production to help your body detox waste and further breakdown food.

The strategy with prebiotics is to include a range of veggies (preferably cooked) and fermentable fibers found in supplements and medicinal foods. Each different type of fiber stimulates the growth of different beneficial bacteria in the gut, so it's important to include all of them as tolerated.

Prebiotic foods and supplements–rotate your fibers on a daily basis;

Prebiotic and starch foods–cooked squashes, cooked carrots, steamed beets, cooked green beans, oats, beans, cooked and cooled potatoes, cooked and cooled white rice, green tipped bananas, and greenish plantains;

Resistant starch–unmodified potato starch, green banana flour, sunfiber, or plantain flour;

Non-starch polysaccharides and soluble fibers–inulin, beta-glucan, FOS, larch arabinogalactan, psyllium husk, pectin, acacia, glucomannan, and flax.

If you find that you feel more bloated, constipated, or experience an increase in gut-related symptoms when you consume fiber, then this is often an indicator of several conditions: first, you have an underlying gut pathology, such as SIBO, mold exposure, or candida, that may need to be addressed; two, you have insufficiency dysbiosis—a low growth of healthy bacteria and diversity; three, your digestive process may not be strong right now. Try lowering your dose—perhaps you can handle half a clove of garlic or half of a sweet potato, but a whole clove might make you gassy, or a whole sweet potato may send your blood sugar or IBS through the roof. It's all about trial and error.

The good news is that just because you may get symptoms when you eat prebiotics, it does not mean they are bad for you; it is simply a sign that your gut and digestive health have some weak links. As you incorporate the Superpowers and customization techniques outlined in this book, you will eventually be better able to tolerate these essential gut superfoods.

Whichever fibers you choose, the *top* benefit of prebiotics is that they increase the production of short-chain fatty acids (SCFAs), which are the real game changers when it comes to a healthy gut ecosystem, even more than probiotics. SCFAs are often called "post-biotics" because they are the by-products created by gut bacteria after they ingest and digest your prebiotics. They boost the acidity of your colon, making it less hospitable to pathogens and more hospitable to the beneficial species of bacteria. SCFAs *also* help to cultivate greater diversity and balance in the biome as a whole, which is perhaps why restrictive eating may seemingly work well in the short term for some folks, only to backfire in the long term, especially if you're not digesting your food well or eating *enough* veggies.

Only one in ten Americans eat even the baseline minimum of three vegetables per day, primarily in the form of tomatoes and potatoes. Short-chain fatty acid concentrations decrease when moderate, balanced carb intake is reduced.

The bottom line is that short-chain fatty acids are *really* what we are going after in terms of consuming prebiotics.

## PROBIOTICS

Last but not least, we cannot talk about prebiotics, fiber, and short-chain fatty acids without discussing probiotics—bacteria found in foods and supplements that mimic the healthy living organisms you naturally have in your microbiome.

Probiotics are nothing new. Humans have been consuming foods like sauerkraut and kimchi (nature's probiotics) for more than 2 million years. Many people's first food, breast milk, is rich in probiotics. Today, you can walk into any grocery store and encounter fifty different options for purchasing probiotics.

Dietary and supplemental probiotics come in several different forms:

- Lactic acid bacterial supplements. These most commonly include different strains from the species *Lactobacillus* and *Bifidobacteria*;
- Soil-based organism supplements: Strains that mimic the types of bacteria our ancestors consumed from the foods they ate in undiluted soil;

- *Saccharomyces cerevisiae* and *Saccharomyces boulardii*: Technically yeasts that are often found in supplements as well; ideal for loose stools and bacterial and fungal overgrowth;
- Fermented foods: Foods with lactic acid-based bacteria and healthy yeasts, cultured for beneficial natural probiotic properties.

Keep in mind, however, that not all probiotics are created equally or work the same. Nor are all probiotics beneficial for all people. In fact, if there is one thing we learned from the American Gut Project—the largest human microbiome research initiative to date, aimed at improving our understanding of the microbial flora involved in human health and disease, it is this: Probiotics and specific bacteria are not the "answer" for human health. Bacterial diversity and abundance is. Even if some probiotics do help, it's been hypothesized that upwards of 90-95 percent of supplemental probiotics sold on store shelves do not contain the probiotics they claim.

The number one reason why this is the case is that most probiotics fail to tell you what strains they use in their formulas. Unfortunately, many supplement companies do not even know themselves what probiotic strains are used in their formulas by the time it makes it to a shelf. Many products also fail to include the strains they use in their formula.

Probiotic naming has three parts to it:

1. Genus (such as *Lactobacillus* or *Bifidobacteria*);
2. Species (such as *Lactobacillus rhamnosus*);
3. Strain (such as *Lactobacillus rhamnosus* GG).

Most probiotics for purchase tell you the genus and species but do not disclose the specific strains used—and there can be dozens of different strains! Strains are like the varying types of Goldendoodle dogs you can choose from when getting a new puppy. There are F1, F1B, F2, and F2B Doodles. These differences make a big difference in terms of the dog's characteristics. F1s, for example, are 50 percent Poodle and 50 percent Golden Retriever or Labrador Retriever, resulting in a larger, curlier dog. F1Bs, on the other hand, are 25 percent Retriever and 75 percent Poodle, and they are the most hypoallergenic dogs. Knowing specific Doodle types allows dog owners to pick the dog that best fits their needs, and the same principle applies to probiotics.

For example, a probiotic label may contain a popular probiotic strain, *Lactobacillus rhamnosus* GG, which has been shown to stop diarrhea in its tracks (79). Another probiotic may also contain *Lactobacillus rhamnosus*, but also a different strain, such as *Lactobacillus rhamnosus* GR-1, connected to maintaining a healthy vagina and preventing biofilm formation, which has nothing to do with diarrhea. Another probiotic may contain *Bifidobacterium bifidum*, but if they do not specify the strain used, such as *Bifidobacterium bifidum* CIDCA 537 or *Bifidobacterium bifidum* CIDCA 5310, you may find that one probiotic *can* inhibit invasion by pathogens like salmonella, whereas the other has no effect at all.

Beyond the lack of probiotic strain transparency, there are several other reasons why not all probiotics are cracked up to be what they claim. Many formulas do not include enough probiotics to make a difference. A therapeutic dose of probiotics includes at least 50 billion CFU (colony-forming units) of bacteria per dose or greater. Probiotics are also highly unstable. Probiotic treatments are packed with bacteria, but once swallowed, their numbers are dramatically diminished by the digestive process, lowering the chances of therapeutic effect. Probiotics are particularly sensitive to stomach acid and bile salts unless manufactured with this in mind. To survive some wear and tear, you want probiotics with at least 50 billion bacterial strains, an appropriate capsule delivery system (such as a slow-release gel capsule), and/or a symbiotic component combined (prebiotics).

Keep in mind, too, that probiotic marketing is clever. Just like "all natural" chicken or "real fruit" fruit gummies, a product that claims to be a "good source of probiotics" is part of the Wild, Wild West of food marketing. One study on commercial yogurts found that you'd have to eat 25 total servings to get the baseline of probiotics promoted on the label. Other research on supplements has revealed similar findings—missing the actual ingredients they claimed. If a product tells you it's legitimate with a "clinically-verified dose" but only has internal studies to prove it (or no studies at all), you may want to think twice.

Also, be aware that not all probiotics work for everyone. Most probiotic companies won't tell you *not* to take their formula. However, if you have an underlying gut pathology, probiotics sometimes may make you feel worse, from skin breakouts to bloating, IBS, headaches, or seemingly no benefit at all.

This can happen for a couple of reasons: one, the formula contains strains of bacteria that you already have enough of; two, the formula is not a quality supplement or does not bypass your stomach or small intestine, where lots of bacteria don't belong; three, you may have an initial healing or adverse reaction as you introduce probiotics to your system. However, if adverse side effects last longer than 7-10 days, then the formula is probably not for you.

Finally, as discussed, probiotics need to be paired with prebiotics in order to actually tick in your gut. When you consume prebiotics, you help multiply your probiotics, so you can increase your beneficial bacteria over time. This is why some companies are now creating symbiotic products—probiotics paired with prebiotics in capsule form.

So, the big question: To probiotic or not probiotic?

Probiotics *can* be beneficial adjuncts to your Total Gut Reset as long as you go with a legitimate strain. I am continually experimenting and updating my top picks in my recommendations for my patients in my programs and always staying on top of the most up-to-date research.

## ABUNDANCE

If there is one thing you have hopefully learned thus far, it is that a happy gut microbiome thrives upon an abundant variety of nutrient-dense foods.

I call this eating with an abundance mindset, thinking "what nutrients can I have" to nourish my body, versus "what can't I have?" An abundance mindset also promotes eating as unrestrictedly as possible.

We all require the consumption of energy in the form of food, air, and water for sustenance and good health. Think of it this way: Your body is a Ferrari. The more quality fuel you put into a Ferrari, and the more often you attend to its needs and maintenance (regular service checks, premium oil), the higher-performing, smooth, and longer it rides. Try to get by on less frequent oil checks and cheap gas? The less efficiently that Ferrari runs and lasts.

Nine times out of ten, the main reason that my clients are frustrated with their metabolism, stubborn body fat, fatigue, bloating, or seasonal allergies is that they are not eating enough or they are bound to restriction. In the pursuit of better gut health, many folks fall victim to avoidant restrictive food intake disorder (ARFID), limiting their eating to only 5-10 foods—not because they fear "getting fat," but because it's all their body can handle. Others innocently get trapped in orthorexia, an unhealthy obsession over eating healthily, as food rule after food rule accumulates over time, and food lists conflict. One low-histamine diet online says avocados are okay, while another says heck no! On the anti-candida diet, red potatoes are fine, but on a specific carbohydrate diet, potatoes are a death sentence.

Remember: Nutrients themselves are a baseline essential for healing. Without nutrients, you have no vitamins, minerals, amino acids, fiber, fatty acids, enzymes, and other compounds to repair your gut lining, feed and cultivate beneficial bacteria, strengthen your immune system, fight free radicals, or supply mitochondria with fuel to create energy for all your cells.

As simple as this sounds, when deciding what to eat for any meal, ask yourself: "How can I nourish my gut bugs with an abundance of nutrients?" Optimally, the body runs best on a diet rich in diversity, moderation, and balance with all three macronutrients: protein, fat, and fiber, plus medicinal doses of probiotic foods.

*All with an 80/20 balance, of course.* Basically, no perfection. Break the rules. I like to challenge my clients to eat a high-quality version of an "imperfect" food at least 1-2 times per week to keep their microbes and mindset flexible. Full permission.

Prepare homemade Mac and cheese with real grass-fed cheddar and brown rice noodles, and throw in some shredded chicken or ground turkey. Eat a scoop of real vanilla ice cream—no funky gums or sweeteners, or bake real chocolate chip cookies with real brown sugar like grandma used to make. Enjoy the grass-fed burger with sweet potato fries or homemade gluten-free pizza at the local mom-and-pop. You get the picture.

A great sign of good gut health, good hormones, peace, and brain health is the ability to tolerate some imperfect foods and not feel wrecked! Like the ability to go out to eat on a Saturday and order something not cooked in pristine oil and be ok. Or the ability to travel and not feel like you have to pack all of your food.

Your body constantly wants to work for you. Not against you. Break a (food) rule.

*Bonus: Total Gut Reset Nutrition Blueprint*

Check out the Total Gut Reset Nutrition Blueprint in the Resources: Eat and Supplement for Your Gut Type section at the back of this book for a complete list of gut-loving foods and meal ideas to feed a happy gut.

# GUT LOVE HABIT 4: NOURISH YOUR GUT BUGS

Eat fat, protein, and fiber (or two or three) at meals—including foods of 2-3 different colors in each (for example, green chard, orange roasted carrots, chicken thighs, and green avocado).

Bonus: Eat 1-2 servings of fermented probiotic foods daily, especially kimchi, sauerkraut, kefir or water kefir, cultured plain yogurt, and fermented vegetables.

Pro tip: Get outside of your box and vary up your foods to nourish your gut bugs. Pick at least 2-3 rotating breakfasts, lunches, and dinners with different nutrients in them. When we eat the same things every day, our body only gets a select amount of nutrients.

## *GUT RESET EXPERIMENT 1:* ***BLOOD SUGAR CHALLENGE***

Balance your blood sugar to balance your gut bugs. In addition to eating balanced meals during the day, dial in the following four "blood sugar balance" hacks for 3-7 days and observe how your energy, cravings, and digestion shift:

**Hack 1:** Consume 20 -30 grams of protein and drink 16-20 ounces of water with sea salt in the first 1-2 hours of waking...Before coffee.

**Hack 2:** At mealtimes, eat your protein, fat, and greens first and your starch last to decrease a blood sugar spike.

**Hack 3:** Cook and cool starches before consuming them to increase resistant starch and decrease the glycemic index (i.e., cooked and cooled potatoes, sweet potatoes, green plantains, gluten-free oatmeal, and rice).

**Hack 4:** For snacks, if you truly are hungry, snack on protein or healthy fat between meals. Eat fruit after a meal, tossed into a smoothie or with healthy fat, like nuts or coconut butter, while sticking to 1-2 small servings per day.

## *GUT RESET EXPERIMENT 2:* ***30 PLANT CHALLENGE***

How many different plant foods do you eat in a week?

Researchers from the American Gut Project found that people regularly eating thirty-plus different types of plant foods per week have a more diverse microbiome than those eating ten or fewer different plant foods a week (remember: A diverse microbiome seems positive, as different bacteria have different effects on our risk of disease).

On that note, take the thirty-plus plant challenge....

Step 1. Take inventory of what different plants you regularly eat in a given week.

See the plant list below. These can include different varieties of the same foods, such as green apples and red apples, orange carrots, and purple carrots, as well as herbs and spices (basil, parsley, oregano, etc.).

Step 2. Make a list of plants to add.

What plants could you add to the mix for the week? The point isn't to get fixated on thirty types; the point is to keep your diet diverse, mix up what you eat, and try to eat a variety of different fruits, veggies, legumes, spices, herbs, some seeds and nuts rather than eating the same ones each day. If you're currently on 12 types and jump to 18, that's a win for your gut!

Step 3. Shop your list.

Hit the store and farmer's market to stock up.

Step 4. Just eat it. Aim for thirty (or ten or fifteen).

Add your plants to recipes, snacks, and daily meals. Do veggies make you bloat? Cook, puree, sauté, juice, steam, mash, chop, or mince 'em and take enzymes and butyrate to aid absorption.

# NOT-SO-BORING VEGGIE IDEAS

Make 'em taste good, gosh darn it! Some ideas include:

- Asparagus: roasted with olive oil, pepper and sea salt, fermented, wrapped in turkey slices;
- Brussels sprouts: sauteed crispy, mixed with turkey bacon, tossed with balsamic vinegar;
- Cauliflower: cauliflower rice seasoned with coconut flakes or coconut aminos, mashed, roasted with sea salt, seasoned with turmeric and ghee;
- Carrots: roasted Rainbow carrots, seasoned with dill & lemon, carrot fries with aioli dipping sauce;
- Green beans: fermented, green bean fries, AIP green bean casserole with coconut milk, wrapped in turkey bacon;
- Greens: lettuce wraps, sautéed in coconut oil and sea salt, mixed greens with paleo dressing;
- Rutabaga, parsnip, and turnips: Fries or chips, roasted with sea salt and olive oil;
- Spaghetti squash: With pesto or melted ghee and sea salt, topped with chicken salad or meatballs or "pizza" meat sauce (ground turkey, olives, basil, olive oil, coconut flakes);
- Sweet potatoes: chips, fries, mashed;
- Winter squash: roasted with cinnamon, topped with cheese sauce, butternut squash bowl, squash "Oatmeal", stuffed acorn squash;
- Zucchini and yellow squash: chips, zoodles, roasted with sea salt and avocado oil;
- Farmer's Surprise: Go to a local farmer's market or natural grocery and buy something in season—fresh herbs, veggies, fresh fruits. Shop "in season" and locally.

# ULTIMATE PLANT FOODS LIST

Plants include not only the food itself but the different varieties of each plant (such as green grapes, red grapes, and purple grapes; baby kale, dino kale, and Tuscan kale; and different herbs and spices).

## VEGGIES

- Acorn squash
- Arrowroot
- Artichoke
- Arugula
- Asparagus
- Bamboo shoots
- Beets
- Beetroot
- Bell pepper
- Bok choy
- Broccoli
- Broccoli rabe
- Brussels sprouts
- Butternut squash
- Cabbage and sauerkraut
- Cauliflower
- Carrots and rainbow carrots
- Cassava
- Chayote
- Celeriac
- Celery
- Chard
- Chicory
- Cucumber
- Collards
- Courgette
- Crookneck squash
- Daikon
- Dandelion greens
- Eggplant
- Fennel
- Ginger root
- Green beans
- Horseradish
- Jicama
- Kale
- Kohlrabi
- Leeks
- Lettuce
- Mushrooms
- Okra
- Onions
- Olives
- Parsnips
- Potatoes
- Pumpkin
- Radicchio
- Radishes
- Rutabagas
- Shallots
- Spaghetti squash
- Spinach
- Spring greens
- Spring
- Squash
- Swedes
- Sweet potato
- Summer squash (yellow squash, zucchini)
- Turnips
- Tomatillo
- Tomatoes
- Yam root
- Water Chestnuts
- Watercress

## FRUITS

- Acai
- Apple
- Avocados
- Bananas
- Blueberries
- Blackcurrants
- Melon
- Cherries
- Coconut
- Cranberry
- Figs
- Grapes

- Kiwi
- Lemon
- Lime
- Mango
- Melons
- Nectarine
- Orange
- Papaya
- Passionfruit
- Peaches
- Pears
- Pineapple
- Plantains
- Plums
- Pomegranate
- Raspberries
- Redcurrants
- Rhubarb
- Strawberries
- Watermelon

## HERBS AND SPICES

- Basil
- Coriander
- Chives
- Cinnamon
- Cumin
- Dill
- Garlic
- Ginger
- Nutmeg
- Oregano
- Paprika
- Parsley
- Pepper
- Rosemary
- Sage
- Thyme
- Turmeric

## PLANT FATS AND OILS

- Avocado oil
- Olive oil
- Coconut oil
- Macadamia oil
- Flax oil
- Hemp seed oil
- Pumpkin seed oil
- Sesame oil

## NUTS AND SEEDS

- Almonds
- Brazil nuts
- Cashews
- Hazelnuts
- Macadamia nuts
- Pecans
- Pistachios
- Chia seeds
- Hemp seeds
- Flaxseed
- Pumpkin seeds
- Sesame seeds
- Sunflower seeds
- Tahini (sesame seed butter)
- Nut butters
- Walnuts

## LEGUMES

- Adzuki beans (red mung bean)
- Black beans
- Black turtle beans
- Black eyed peas
- Baked beans
- Butter beans
- Black-eyed peas
- Cannellini beans
- Chickpeas (and hummus)
- Fava beans

- Green peas
- Kidney beans
- Lentils—black, red, green, yellow, brown
- Mung beans
- Navy beans
- Peanuts
- Pinto beans
- Split peas
- Yellow peas

## SPECIFIC PREBIOTIC, COLONIC, AND SHORT-CHAIN FATTY ACID FOODS

### FRUCTOOLIGOSACCHARIDES (FRUCTANS):

- Garlic
- Onions
- Leeks
- Chicory root
- Jerusalem artichoke
- Dandelion greens
- Burdock root
- Honey
- Greenish bananas
- Asparagus
- Rye flour
- Barley
- Burdock root
- FOS supplements (especially inulin)

### GALACTO-OLIGOSACCHARIDES (GALACTANS):

- Beans
- Lentils
- Jerusalem artichoke
- GOS supplements

### BETA-GLUCANS (COLONIC FOODS):

- Mushrooms
- Dates
- Oats (gluten-free)
- Seaweed
- Algae
- Spirulina

### PECTINS (COLONIC FOODS):

- Fruits (especially peaches, apples, pears, oranges, grapefruit, apricots)
- Potato
- Peas
- Carrots
- Parsnips
- Green beans
- Legumes

## POLYPHENOLS (COLONIC FOODS):

- Apples
- Artichokes
- Berries
- Black and green tea
- Black currants
- Cherries
- Cloves
- Cocoa
- Dark chocolate
- Dark leafy greens
- Herbal tea
- Nuts
- Plums

## RESISTANT STARCH (COLONIC FOODS):

- Cooked and cooled potatoes
- Cooked and cooled parboiled rice
- Cooked and cooled oats
- Cooked and cooled legumes and lentils (soaked or sprouted)
- Green plantains and dehydrated plantain chips
- Green-tipped bananas
- Cassava

## SOLUBLE FIBER (COLONIC FOODS):

- Cooked and softened tubers and root vegetables (rutabaga, turnips, radish, carrots, beets)
- Summer squash
- Winter squash
- Pumpkin
- Berries

## PREBIOTIC SUPPLEMENTS:

- *Supplements are generally better digested by people with bloating, SIBO, IBS, and candida*
- Acacia fiber (may be used as an alternative to psyllium husk)
- Beta-glucan, or β-glucan
- Chicory root
- Fructo-oligosaccharides
- Galacto-oligosaccharides
- Glucomannan
- Inulin

- Partially hydrolyzed guar gum*
- Pectin*
- Psyllium husk powder*
- Resistant starch (potato starch, green-banana flour, unmodified plantain flour, arrowroot starch)*

### SHORT CHAIN FATTY ACIDS:

- 5-9 servings of vegetables per day
- 1-2 servings of fruits per day
- Grass-fed butter and ghee
- Resistant starches (green bananas, plantains, and banana flour; cooked and cooled beans, lentils, potatoes, rice, muesli)
- Supplements ( butyrate, propionate, and acetate)

## THE BOTTOM LINE

The food you eat can change your gut microbiome. Eighty percent of the time, eat real, gut-loving proteins, fats, and fiber. For the other 20 percent of the time, let life happen.

# CHAPTER 15:
# SUPERPOWER 5: REST

"I'll sleep when I'm dead!" This was my top phrase when I first started my business.

Based on what I know now, allow me to rephrase: *Not* sleeping will kill you (and your healthy gut bugs) faster.

Sleep is a panacea, a remedy when it comes to optimal health. It's the time when the body and brain detox, recover, rebuild, and restore. If sleep is cut short, the body and brain don't have time to complete all the phases needed for muscle and organ repair, memory consolidation, the release of hormones regulating growth and appetite, detoxification, and microbial balance.

## THE SECRET TO MAKING A MILLION BUCKS

Josh didn't have time to sleep.

As an entrepreneur running a mid-size brand strategy business, a member of two other company boards, the creator of a side-gig tech start-up, a CrossFit junkie, and the father of two little girls under the age of two, sleep was the last thing on his agenda. He averaged at most 4-5 hours of sleep most nights over the past ten years. Even when he did sleep, he never slept all the way through the night, often waking up once or twice, at least, to go to the bathroom or with a racing idea in his mind.

Although his brain was able to keep going and going, his body wasn't. Chronic allergies, recurring sinus infections and strep throat, an annoying twitch and watering in his right eye, and occasional stabbing pains in his chest brought him to my office after seeing seven other doctors and two ER visits that resulted in no diagnosis.

"I've had brain scans, chest scans, a colonoscopy, allergy shots, and seven rounds of antibiotics," he told me. "Nothing seems to work."

Upon reviewing his food and poo log, his stack of supplements, and his daily schedule, I discovered that he was doing all the things, like so many others.

"But how are you sleeping?" I asked.

"Not great. But not horrible. I've always been a short-term sleeper—four to five hours—and functioned fine. I think I'm just one of those people who can run on little to no sleep. Maybe I'm just missing some sort of vitamin in my diet? Or do I need to take a different probiotic?"

I challenged him: "This week, I don't want you to change your habits except for one thing: Sleep. Try to candle down at night—shut off your screens two to three hours before bed. Turn the Wi-Fi off on your phone. Stay in bed for at least six and maybe even seven hours, in a pitch-black, cool room. Just focus on sleep."

Fast forward six months and Josh was a completely new person: no more weird eye twitches or chest pains; sinus infection and antibiotic-free for months; better control of his allergies; Turbo energy, and he was sleeping seven to seven-and-a-half hours a night.

"I never knew how good I could feel until I felt.. well... good!" he told me at a monthly check-in.

One year later, Josh's tech side gig had become his new hustle—but he wasn't hustling nearly as hard as he had all those years he went without sleep. Even better, his little start-up company netted over $1.1 million in the first year, and his work-life balance continued to go through the roof.

Sleep—quality sleep—is essential in helping you and your gut bugs feel good.

## SLEEP DEPRIVATION SIDE EFFECTS

Sleep deprivation *decreases* beneficial bacteria. In a study of healthy, young, normal-weight men with no sleep disorders and regular eating patterns, scientists found that with two nights of sleeping less than 6 hours, the men experienced a significant decrease in beneficial bacteria and an increase in bacteria linked to insulin sensitivity, cravings, obesity, and type 2 diabetes. This means that, after just 1-2 days of no sleep, your gut decreases its ability to properly metabolize glucose, feel satisfied, and naturally resist food cravings while decreasing leptin.

As for detoxification, your glymphatic system—the part of the lymphatic system that removes toxic wastes from your central nervous system, specifically your brain—is ten times more active during sleep. Hence, if you don't get enough sleep, you risk a build-up of toxins in the brain, which impacts your nervous system (stress pathways) and Gut-Brain Connection.

Cognitively, sleeping less than 6 hours per night results in the same cognitive function and alertness as a person with a blood alcohol concentration of 0.05%—legally drunk.

Sleep loss also negatively affects mood and emotional processing, leading to significantly higher subjective experiences of stress due to a 50 percent increase in cortisol levels—from road rage during rush hour traffic to frustration while reading an email or feeling annoyed at the funny look that guy just gave you.

So, how amazing is your sleep?

Unfortunately, more than one in three Americans are sleep deprived, and one in four experience insomnia on a regular basis, meaning they wake in the middle of the night. Even if you don't experience insomnia, many people's circadian rhythms are out of whack—leaving them unable to get quality sleep despite *trying* to sleep.

## WHY WE CAN'T SLEEP

Sleep deprivation does *not* typically happen because we don't want to sleep. For many people, it's because they *can't* sleep.

The reason? You guessed it! Gut health and stress.

In an ideal world, our bodies would "rise" and "set" with the sun. For the vast majority of our ancestors' evolutionary history, we lived in peace and harmony with the natural rhythms of day and night, with no exposure to artificial light included. Humans were physically active throughout the day and rested at night.

Today, our lives are not in sync with the way our circadian rhythms are designed to function. We look at screens for upwards of 12 hours per day. We are stuck indoors with little fresh air and artificial lights during the day, and we use bright, artificial light at night. We drink, on average, 2 to 3 cups of coffee per day or chug energy drinks—telling our body clocks to keep going. We eat late into the evening or skip breakfast and intermittently fast early in the day when our digestive fire is highest. We hit the gym after work, during the time of day when our body's clock is beginning to wind down. Our biological clocks are greatly affected by signals from the environment, especially light and darkness, as well as high-stress demands, whether from the caffeine jolt of a double espresso latte or the rigors of an intense CrossFit workout at 7 p.m.

Microbes and circadian genes are inextricably intertwined. Studies show that circadian clock misalignment–achieved through eating, working, working out, or looking at screens at the wrong times–and sleep deprivation affect circadian clock gene expression and our microbial community structure. Your gut bacteria change location within the gut, as well as change their short-chain fatty acid outputs over the course of 24 hours in a day. If your sleep is off, then your biome's clock gets off too, which may help explain why the prevalence of metabolic syndrome—a by-product of gut dysbiosis—is higher in shift workers and in people who often experience jet lag.

In addition, levels of the hormone cortisol *should* look like a bell curve—they spike up first thing in the morning, peak mid-day, and gradually dip in the evening up to bedtime. However, if your body is living in a constant state of stress or inflammation during the day, normal cortisol patterns also get out of whack, making you wake up. In folks who experience insomnia, particularly between the hours of 2 a.m. and 5 a.m., blood sugar and cortisol imbalances are typically to blame.

If you wake up at 2 or 3 a.m., the likely culprit is blood sugar. When blood sugar goes too low (hypoglycemia), cortisol *also* drops, and the body sends out alarm signals—sweating, jitteriness, heart palpitations, anxiety—in the form of adrenaline. You feel wired and tired at the same time, wanting to sleep but unable to. Your body is too wound up.

This pattern of waking is common in people with dysbiosis—gut bacteria that have not absorbed and digested food appropriately. It's also common in those who eat low-fat, low-protein, or higher sugar and carbohydrate-based diets, as well as those who have had alcohol in the evening. Alcohol causes blood sugar to rise and then drop off suddenly within a 1 to 3 hour span. For this reason, folks with hypoglycemic and low cortisol episodes find that a small protein-based snack before bed can be helpful for sleeping through the night, such as a cup of bone broth, organic cottage cheese, Greek yogurt, leftover protein from dinner, or some quality protein powder shaken up in water, almond milk, or coconut milk.

If you tend to wake up closer to the 4 a.m. or 5 a.m. time frame, the HPA axis and cortisol itself, rather than the blood-sugar-cortisol relationship, is more likely the culprit. You're most commonly feeling wired as if it's time to start the day, even though your alarm hasn't gone off yet. This can happen due to ongoing inputs of stress throughout the day and evening hours—from watching TV and using screens late at night, imbalanced diets or poor absorption of nutrients, high caffeine intake, and other circadian rhythm imbalances.

Some helpful tactics for *staying* asleep during the wee morning hours in order to get a full night's sleep include keeping your bedroom cool—68 degrees or below—throughout the night. Coolness supports both sleep onset and maintenance since your body temperature rises as sleep goes on throughout the night. Also, ensure there is absolute darkness in the room. I recommend covering or removing any glowing things from the bedroom, investing in blackout blinds, or using a sleep mask. Some supplements, like melatonin, CBD oil, or adrenal adaptogens, such as Ashwagandha and Rhodiola, can also be helpful, but it's important to know that customization is key.

For example, I've seen boatloads of clients who take high doses of melatonin to try to sleep better, only to find their insomnia worsens. Melatonin hormone deficiency only accounts for a small percentage of poor sleep cases and is best used by those with poor sleep onset. And like all hormones, it's important to treat it with respect. High-dose melatonin may turn down your body's natural melatonin production–which can exacerbate nighttime waking in the long run. With melatonin, less really is more, like 3 mg of delayed-release formula. Lastly, for quality sleep throughout the night, supporting your gut health cannot be overlooked. Prebiotics and probiotics have been shown to positively affect the quality of your non-REM and REM sleep,[1] along with inflammation reduction, also suggesting that a happy, healthy microbe could be the "sleep drug" we've all been needing.

## IDEAL SLEEP

Better sleep and a better biome are a two-way street. The better our sleep (and the better our circadian clock), the healthier and more diverse our gut biome, and the more diverse and healthier our gut biome, the better our sleep. Most adults need between 7 and 9 hours of sleep each night (Six *if* you have the special gene mutation that allows you to function normally with just 4 to 6 hours of sleep a night).

Quality sleep is best achieved when we optimize our circadian rhythms *throughout the day*. Understanding the Chinese Medicine Clock is a great way to do this.

1 https://www.frontiersin.org/articles/10.3389/fnbeh.2016.00240/full

# YOUR CHINESE MEDICINE CLOCK RHYTHMS

The Chinese Medicine clock is a great roadmap for helping your body get "back online" if your circadian rhythms are off. According to Chinese medicine, your body has a natural time of day when one system is working the hardest, and different times of day are best for eating, sleeping, thinking, creating, and working. On the flip side, if you find yourself feeling out of balance at a certain time of day, it can also signal an imbalance physically, mentally, and/or emotionally.

Think of your circadian rhythm clock as a roadmap to guide you toward syncing up with your body's natural rhythms.

## MORNING

**3-5 a.m.: Sleep soundly.**
**Organ: Lung hour.**
**Actions:**

- If you happen to wake up between these hours, gentle breathing exercises can boost balance.

**Emotions being processed:** Grief and sadness.

**5-7 a.m.: Do the do, drink warm lemon water, and move your body.**
**Organ: Large intestine hour.**
**Actions:**

- Waking up and releasing is key during these hours;
- Sometimes, you may run into constipation issues if you wake up on the earlier side of this window since your body is still in cleansing mode;
- Encourage elimination by taking time to do the do, drinking 16 ounces of warm lemon water, and moving your body with an energizing workout;
- Physically moving and releasing internal excess also assists with your emotions.

**Emotions being processed:** Guilt, stagnation.

**7-9 a.m.: Eat a grounding, easy-to-digest breakfast.**
**Organ: Stomach.**
**Actions:**

- Your body is ready to digest during the "stomach" hour, but hold off on the quick-digesting cereal, bagel, fruit, or granola bar;
- Ground your body (and blood sugar) for the day ahead with some sustainable, hearty protein, along with healthy fats and cooked vegetables;
- Add in digestive enzymes and HCl (hydrochloric acid) if you need extra support;
- Warm tea is also a winner in place of iced coffee, cold drinks, or even hot coffee. Warm herbal tea stimulates the stomach's natural warming functions and does not impact stress levels as coffee and caffeine do.

**Emotions being processed:** Despair.

**9-11 a.m.: Do creative, mentally challenging work.**
**Organs: Pancreas and spleen.**
**Actions:**

- Thinking, creating, and working is the name of the game in the mid-morning hours when your spleen and pancreas transmute your protein-rich breakfast into usable energy.

**Emotions being processed:** Jealousy, worry, low self-esteem.

## AFTERNOON

**11 a.m.-1 p.m.: Eat a light Lunch, take a recess**
**Organ: Heart**
**Actions:**

- Your body works hard, pumping blood to your heart;
- To let it do its due diligence, eat "lunch for a queen" (unlike breakfast for a "king");
- Put a little spark of joy into the day—take a recess for a yoga class or workout if you didn't start your day with a full routine, meet up with friends or co-workers for lunch, take a stroll outside for some fresh air, and break free from your screens.

**Emotions being processed:** Joy or frightful sadness.

**1-3 p.m.: Check off your detail-oriented tasks.**
**Organ: Small intestine.**
**Actions:**

- Your body does some of its strongest "gut work" (since your small intestine is the longest organ in your digestive tract);

- This is also the most common time that people experience indigestion and bloating (a reason to eat a lighter lunch);
- This is the best time of day to do your checklist and detail-oriented tasks—such as blasting through those emails, crunching the chores, separating the good from bad, and organizing;
- Do things that need to get done but don't require tons of brain power while your body is focusing hard on digestion.

**Emotions being processed:** Insecurity (perhaps linked with the higher occurrence of gas and bloating during this time).

**3-5 p.m.: Cortisol and energy dip.**
**Organ: Bladder.**
**Actions:**

- Cortisol and blood sugar levels generally dip in the afternoon, especially if you have HPA D. Considering this time frame is also the bladder hour, and the kidneys that activate the bladder are connected to your adrenal glands, it makes sense;
- To combat the mid-day dip, snack on something with sea salt or add a pinch—up to 1 teaspoon—into a tall glass of water. Salt acts like an emergency brake for the cortisol dip (since cortisol zaps up sodium reserves);
- Consider standing up or sitting on a yoga ball for work if you sit at a desk (to keep from falling asleep);
- Balance blood sugar with a protein and/or fat-based snack, and avoid carbohydrates, sugar, and coffee.

**Emotions being processed:** Irritation, moving energy internally.

**5-7 p.m.: Wind-down mode.**
**Organ: Kidney.**
**Actions:**

- The work day is done or winding down, and chances are you're feeling mentally and perhaps physically spent. This is the perfect time to replenish vital energy. For some, this may mean connecting with friends, a gentle movement session (yoga, a walk, or a workout), getting some fresh air, or putting your feet up. The average population tends to gravitate towards TV, cocktails, or more sitting post-work, but be cautious of how these activities can actually be more draining and less restorative, especially if you've been sitting all day long or if alcohol is consumed several days per week, which is more toxic for the kidneys than nourishing.

**Emotions being processed:** Fear.

## EVENING:

**7-9 p.m.: Self-care, connection with loved ones.**
**Organ: Pericardium (supports your heart function).**
**Action:**

- More building upon self-care, restoration, and connection. This is the time to share a meal with friends or loved ones or simply nourish yourself with a nutrient-dense meal;
- Attend a social gathering for a sense of genuine connection;
- Continue to restore—a hot shower, face mask, book reading, daydreaming, a creative outlet, yoga flow, gentle stretching, meditation, or anything that builds into your own sense of well being;
- The key take home: Nourish the heart and rejuvenate the body after a long day.

**Emotions being processed:** Excessive euphoria and compassion.

**9-11 p.m.: Candle down**
**Organ: Metabolism, lymphatic system (drainage system)**
**Action:**

- Relaxation continues—but with a key emphasis on candling down for circadian clock optimization, in line with what your metabolism is also craving at this time—relaxation;
- After working hard all day, your body is officially in candle-down mode, greatly influenced by the darkness of the night;
- Screens, bright artificial lights, and blue light exposure can be overstimulating to the circadian clock and central nervous system, impeding metabolic optimization and lymphatic detoxification;
- Shut the screens off, use a lamp or candlelight, sip warm tea, read a good book, journal, meditate, stretch, and perhaps even get to bed!
- Gold standard HPA axis goal: 10 p.m. bedtime.

**Emotions being processed:** Hopelessness and confusion.

**11 p.m.-1 a.m.: Sleepytime.**
**Organ: Gallbladder**
**Action:**

- Regenerating is the name of the game—especially as your gallbladder goes to work.
- The gallbladder works to support the liver in detoxification, excrete bile (waste), and digest healthy fats;

- If you're not resting by 11 p.m., you could have issues with digestion as well as emotional components of decision-making since this time frame is also connected to indecisiveness and resentment (read: text messages you regret sending at midnight). Nothing good happens after 10 p.m.

**Emotions being processed:** Indecisiveness and resentment.

**1-3 a.m.: Detox, blood sugar balance, cortisol restoration time.**
**Organ: Liver.**
**Action:**

- Ideally, you are in deep sleep and dream mode between 1 and 3 a.m. However, if you find yourself waking up to pee, eat a snack, or for no reason at all, it could mean something is not quite right "under the hood."
- Your liver is at its peak hour—working hard to detox toxins and wastes that have built up in the body from the day. Translation: That coffee, glass of wine, or chocolate cake you ate for dessert may be waking you up.
- In addition, your liver is the main organ responsible for storing and utilizing glucose (i.e., sugar from food), secreting bile acids and digestive enzymes, *and* "feeding cortisol" with glucose. However, if your HPA axis is stressed, then your liver goes into overdrive trying to keep up with the demands of blood sugar imbalance and cortisol as you sleep;
- Often, insomnia or waking up in the middle of the night can be a sign of blood sugar levels dropping and both cortisol and adrenaline kicking in as your body's emergency brake to keep you alive;
- Anxiety during these hours may also wake you up.

**Emotions being processed:** Anger, anxiety, frustration.

## GUT LOVE HABIT #5: GET YOUR BEAUTY SLEEP

Sleep for 7-9 hours each night in a cool (68 degrees or below) pitch-dark room (use blackout curtains, an eye mask, and remove electronics and lights). In the evenings, put your phone in another room or airplane mode 2-3 hours before bed.

Pro Tip: If you struggle with insomnia, try these hacks at bedtime:

- Shut off screens 1-2 hours before bed;
- Read, meditate, create, or journal instead;
- Eat a small protein snack before bed if you ate an early dinner (try bone broth, coconut yogurt, additive-free protein powder);
- Drink a cup of Bedtime or Sleepy Time tea;
- Supplement with magnesium glycinate or magnesium citrate in the evening; or low-dose, slow-release melatonin (1-3 mg);
- In the evenings, put your phone in another room or put it in airplane mode 2-3 hours before bed.

## GUT RESET EXPERIMENT: RESET YOUR CIRCADIAN RHYTHMS

Your body's natural cleansing rhythms happen on a biological clock. According to Chinese medicine, your body has a natural time of day when one system is working the hardest. Carve out one day to devote 100% effort to following an ideal circadian rhythm schedule.

### *EXAMPLE RHYTHM RESET:*

**5-7 a.m.: Wake up.** "Ground" yourself by stepping outside for fresh air and morning sun; Morning routine—meditation, prayer, plan to workout early in the day or afternoon—especially if you have a tough time falling asleep at night.
**7-9 a.m.: Breakfast.** Limit coffee to one cup of quality (organic) coffee per day, after food.
**9-12 p.m.: Mentally taxing tasks.** Creative flow.
**12-2 p.m.: Mid-day break & Lunch.** Walk. Change scenery. Workout. Yoga class. Meditation. Eat low starch, moderate protein, fats, and veggies.
**2-5 p.m.: Detail-oriented tasks & small snack.** Planning, emails, logistics, checklist, to-dos. Small snack if needed. Something with protein and/or sea salt, like a grass-fed beef jerky, a handful of macadamia nuts, or leftover chicken salad with sea salt; avoid sugar.
**5-7 pm: Post-work break.** Something social or with family. Movement. Evening walk.
**6-8 p.m.: Simple supper.** Starchy tuber or root veggie, protein, greens. Eat your last meal 2-3 hours before bedtime.

**8-11 p.m.: Evening wind down.** Focus on self-care. Shut screens off 2-3 hours before bed or wear orange-tinted glasses if looking at screens. Hot shower. Read a book instead or connect with loved ones.
**10-11 p.m.: Bed.** Peace out.

Keep a food, mood, and poo log for the day to track how you feel, as well as to note any epiphanies you have.

## THE BOTTOM LINE

Sleep is essential to the health of your body and brain. It's the time when the body and brain detox, recover, rebuild, and restore. If sleep is cut short, so is your organ repair, memory, hormones, energy, appetite cues, detoxification, and digestion.

# CHAPTER 16: SUPERPOWER 6: MOVEMENT

Movement is to the body like sunshine is to a plant.

A plant needs water and rich soil to survive and thrive (just like you need water and nutrient-dense food to survive and thrive), but a plant also needs sunshine to grow and stay strong—just like you need movement to stay strong.

## LESSONS FROM OUR ANCESTORS (AGAIN)

There is a mismatch between our ancestral and modern lifestyles in terms of physical activity. Our natural movement today is almost as big a mismatch as our diet. We no longer eat like our ancestors ate, and we no longer move like our ancestors moved.

Humans living in both prehistoric and contemporary hunter-gatherer societies moved around a lot and were very active, walking approximately ten thousand steps a day. By comparison, the average American walks about 5,000-7,000 steps per day.

Humans *also* moved—they did not formally exercise. Movement was a way of life and not something they over-analyzed or had to convince themselves to do. After all, we are *human beings*, and part of being human is being an active participant in life.

The humans of yesteryear did not know the difference between lifting a heavy log ten times versus deadlifting a barbell ten times, nor did they know the difference between running from a lion or a bear versus running on a treadmill at Orangetheory to burn 500 calories. They simply moved.

## THE GUT MICROBIOME AND EXERCISE

Regular exercise, even just walking and hiking, and a better fitness level promotes better digestion and greater gut microbiota diversity—which, as you know by now, is correlated with better health overall. Exercise powerfully decongests internal organs, stimulates circulation, flushes your lymphatic system, reduces inflammatory cytokines, decreases the abundance of pathogenic microbes, *and* increases short-chain fatty acids.

By default, the more diverse your gut is, the better an athlete you can become. If your microbiome is more diverse, it processes the food you eat more efficiently, producing better performance and mitochondria. One study showed an active, "athletic" microbiome supports a higher turnover of carbohydrates, suggesting that people who workout are more likely to have bacteria that better regulate insulin and digest their food—particularly carbs—better. Another trial took 37 cancer survivors who were one year post-treatment and put them through a ten-day fitness intervention in which they worked out at a Barry's Bootcamp level intensity. Their beneficial bacteria and diversity increased by 25 percent in as little as ten days, according to their stool samples. One more study in 18 lean and 14 obese sedentary adults found that exercising just 30 to 60 minutes three times per week resulted in an increase in anti-inflammatory gut microbes. Similarly, researchers found that the gut reverted back to its prior state after another six weeks of sedentary behavior. Hence, people who take up exercise do not gain a *permanently* changed microbiome. As long as they are exercising, the gut bacteria changes, just like while you're taking probiotics, you have some beneficial changes, but after 48 hours of stopping a probiotic, you don't see that effect anymore. Nevertheless, exercise is effective at positively changing your gut microbiome, as long as you don't overdo it.

## OVERTRAINING CONUNDRUM

We often hear a lot about how bad sedentary lifestyles are for us—born out by facts such as Americans sitting for an average of 12 hours per day and that sedentary lifestyles make us fat. But we rarely hear about the negative consequences of moving *too* much.

Overtraining appears to have the opposite effect of healthy exercise. Increasing the intensity, frequency, and/or duration of your workout increases your risk of gut inflammation and dysbiosis.

Up to 50 percent of athletes, known for high training intensity most days per week, have been shown to have increased LPS (lipopolysaccharides)—an endotoxic chemical—correlated with leaky gut syndrome. Moreover, in a study of 29 highly trained male triathletes, researchers discovered that, upon competition, 93 percent reported digestive disturbances, and two participants even had to abandon the race because of severe vomiting and diarrhea. Overheating and restricted or reduced blood flow with constant stress can cause a loosening of the tight junctions during intense exercise, pooling blood away from the GI tract to periphery muscles and organs such as the heart and lungs during intense physical activity. Constipation is another common finding in folks who exercise a lot, especially because your body can become mineral and water depleted quickly, even if you're not overheated. Disruption of the brain-gut axis through increased stress also sends "stress" signals to your gut, stalling GI motility. It's a snowball effect.

Exercise also *positively* stimulates the release of hormones and chemicals such as GABA, cortisol, adrenaline, and dopamine—all of which help your body respond to stress by increasing your heart and respiratory rates and turning on the fight or flight mode to help you run faster or jump higher. Dopamine also boosts your internal motivation and mood-boosting chemicals that make finishing an intense marathon, killer CrossFit WOD, or one-rep max back squat more rewarding.

*However*, if these stress-combating hormones and compounds are constantly being released, day in and day out, then they become *detrimental*, allowing for oxidative stress to take over. Your body stays in fight or flight mode. Your performance decreases. You feel lethargic or fatigued, even though you don't want to admit it. Your immune function decreases. Digestive distress arises. High levels of dopamine can also make you more addicted to exercise or related incentives, like snacking, binging, or drinking caffeine and pre-workout drinks.

Additionally, our mental intention and approach to exercise (militant vs. joy-filled) may also play a role in how our gut microbiota responds. One study found that forced treadmill running exacerbates unhealthy gut bacteria and intestinal inflammation, while *voluntary* and enjoyable running diminishes inflammatory cytokines in the colon. So, what do you think happens if overtraining and forced training continues day in and day out? *Inflammation*.

Like all other types of stressors, *not* all stress is bad. Exercise is a positive stressor—particularly for the purposes of elimination—but you want to adopt the "Goldilocks approach" of choosing not too much and not too little.

According to research, the tipping point for gut issues seems to be exercising for two or more hours at 60 percent VO2 maximum. This would mean that a person is exercising at 60 percent of their maximum capacity to utilize oxygen—a moderately intense rate. Other research shows that repetitive strenuous exercise—going hard most days, even if for less than 2 hours, does funky things to your gut bacteria and gut lining. Strenuous exercise, whether it seems like it or not, is a stressor on our bodies. Like any stressor, it elevates levels of our stress hormone cortisol, weakening the tight junctions in the intestinal cell walls and stomping out healthy gut bugs.

This doesn't mean that you should *never* engage in tough or strenuous exercise, nor avoid exercise completely if you struggle with GI issues. However, it's vital to be aware of what strenuous exercise means for you and the potential digestive and microbiota risks that can result from pushing yourself too hard, too frequently, *or* too long.

## DEFINING STRENUOUS EXERCISE

Finding your "just right" amount of exercise stress is like lifting weights or working out for the first time. A hike or power walk might be strenuous if you're out of shape, but if you're a seasoned athlete, a power walk would be more like a cakewalk. In the weight room, to get stronger, you need to add some weight to the bar. However, say your one-rep max bench press is 105 pounds. To warm up, you start off with 65 pounds for five reps, then 85 pounds for another five reps. Then, you move on to 95 pounds for three reps before you finally increase it to 105 pounds, and uh-oh. Eventually, the positive stressor becomes negative—you can't lift it, lift it very well, or you risk injury. Too much of a good thing is not a good thing for your biome or body, and there is no need to push yourself past your limit.

The easiest way to quantify what's strenuous for your body is to do the good ol' Gut Check Method. Around your workouts, ask yourself these three questions:

*How do I feel?*
*Why do I feel this way?*
*What do I need?*

You should feel challenged but not completely wrecked by your workouts. If you're into numbers, you can calculate your maximum heart rate (MHR) or track your HRV (heart rate variability) as a gauge.

To calculate your MHR, subtract your age from 220. So if you're 40 years old, you would subtract 40 from 220 to get an MHR of 180. That means 180 beats per minute is theoretically the maximum number of times your heart should beat while exercising. A strenuous exercise is one that uses 70-85 percent of that maximum rate. The "gut loving" zone—60 percent—would be more like 108 beats per minute or a little less.

## GUT LOVE HABIT 6

Move your body daily in some way, whether you have 7 or 60 minutes. Walking is a great start if you don't already have an exercise routine. Already exercising? Try something new this week, like a new class, sport, gym, trainer, or app outside your usual routine to mix it up.

*Pro Tip: Strength/weights, yoga, HIIT (Bootcamp, circuit, sprints, CrossFit style training), and hiking/walking are the best bets for your microbiome. Long-distance running, chronic cardio, and stationary cardio can diminish gut bacteria diversity and abundance over time if done repetitively.*

## GUT RESET EXPERIMENT: RESTORE

Build in recovery. Incorporate 1-2 *intentional* recovery days each week to recover well. You can still move and sweat—just dial back the intensity. *Recovery day ideas:*

- Manual muscle therapy (dry needling, active release therapy, massage, STIM);
- Lacrosse ball, foam roller, or mobility work;
- Hot-cold therapy (hot cold shower or ice bath plus a sauna after a workout; always start with hot and end with cold, unless you plan to go to sleep afterward, in which case you should end with heat;
- Warm bubble bath with Epsom Salt and/or aromatherapy containing chamomile and lavender;
- Active rest (walk, low-intensity movement, bodyweight workout—cooling off the high-intensity training);
- A yoga or hike day (in place of a workout day);
- Castor oil packs for your muscles and body after workouts;
- Vinyasa, yin, or Hatha flow yoga;
- Tai chi;
- Nature walks;
- Grounding (getting some fresh air, sunshine, and bare feet on the ground).

## TRACK YOUR HEART RATE VARIABILITY

Have you ever wondered what the health impact of a stressful day was? Will you perform well during your 5 a.m. workout tomorrow morning? Is there anything you can do today that would improve your ability to have more energy the next day?

Heart Rate Variability (HRV) may be the piece of data that could help you answer these questions. Heart rate variability is a measure of the variability in heartbeat interval—the amount of time between heartbeats. HRV shows how stressed or relaxed and strong your body's autonomic nervous system (vagus nerve) is.

*Ideally*, we want a higher HRV (more variability or longer time between heartbeats). The higher our HRV, the more likely our cortisol levels (stress hormones) and our vagus nerve are healthy. Low HRV (meaning there is little variability in the space between heartbeats and/or our heartbeats are faster) can point to poor general fitness, high stress levels, lack of sleep, illness, or overtraining—the more likely our body is in fight-or-flight mode.

## *HOW TO TRACK HRV*

Thanks to technology, you can track your HRV at home with a heart rate monitor or device and daily log.

**Step 1. Get a Heart Rate Monitor or Tracker:**
Recommended HRV Trackers:

- HRV4Training (an iOS-only app that measures HRV using the camera and flash on your phone – you simply place your index finger directly over the lens and breathe naturally);
- Simple Heart Rate Monitor and App (ex. BioForce HRV, and Elite HRV work);
- Body Battery by Garmin;
- Oura Ring;
- Whoop Band;

**Step 2: Track Daily Upon Waking for Seven Days to Find Your Baseline:**
No matter the app, the basic premise is the same: Measure HRV once per day, ideally upon waking up.

**Step 3: Review Results and Establish Your Baseline:**
Over time, as data accumulates in the app's log, you'll identify your baseline. Your daily score isn't terribly important; you'll be more interested in seeing how your day-to-day HRV compares with this baseline.

Important note: There aren't normative values of 'good' and 'bad." Instead, use HRV as an individualized biofeedback tool (everyone's HRV is unique to them). If your score is *within* your baseline range or higher, it may be a good day to stick to your workout or even push yourself a bit. If it falls below baseline, it may be a better idea to scale back your training plans or take a rest day.

## THE BOTTOM LINE

What you do with your body is just as important as what you put into it for optimal gut function. Incorporate plenty of lifestyle movement (walking, standing), complimented by a blend of strength training, HIIT, low-intensity aerobics, mobility, and recovery to optimize your biome. Ultimately, *move, don't exercise*, and do things you enjoy. Your body doesn't know the difference between lifting a heavy log ten times versus deadlifting a barbell.

# CHAPTER 17:
# SUPERPOWER 7: DETOX

"Detox" is code for boosting your body's ability to rid itself of wastes and toxins, a daily necessity for a healthy gut.

Have you ever wondered why some days you feel like you're on the mountaintop, and other days, for no apparent reason, you feel sluggish, depressed, and weak?

Chances are, on the days that you don't feel great your body can't handle its toxic load. Simply put: It is poisoned because your detox system, i.e., your elimination pathways, is not up to the task of protecting your body from the toxins you are exposed to.

A total body detox simply entails **intentionally supporting and strengthening your eight cleansing channels:** your skin, lungs, kidneys, colon, liver, gallbladder, lymph, and blood. These eight pathways work hard to keep out the bad guys.

For example: your **skin** acts like body armor, protecting you from many toxins trying to enter the body in the first place, as well as releasing toxins through sweat from your pores.

Your **lungs** exhale carbon dioxide from your bloodstream and breathes oxygen in—helping maintain a neutral and peaceful environment inside.

Your **kidneys** and **colon** flush and release toxins through urine and stool.

Your **liver** is also responsible for assisting in the process of digestion. The liver double-checks your daily food sources to ensure you only get the essential nutrients out of your broccoli or salmon, without the unwanted pesticides or mercury that may have snuck in. Throughout your lifetime, your liver is constantly on the alert to keep as many bad guys out of your body as possible, performing a natural liver cleanse on a daily basis in conjunction with the bacteria that assist in the breakdown of ingested toxins, molecules, pathogens, and medications.

Your **gallbladder** plays backup to the liver, releasing bile that the liver has created, full of wastes and toxins, and excreting it from the body.

Your **lymphatic system**—the fluids in your body—and **bloodstream** carry wastes, cellular trash, and toxins to the liver for processing—your body's main detox site, a natural garbage disposal or cleansing system.

Suppose your body is overloaded with too many toxins to process or your gut bacteria are out of whack. In that case, a domino effect ensues, leading to clogged elimination pathways and all the side effects that go with it: fatigue, constipation, dehydration, bloating, brain fog, headaches, hormonal imbalances, food sensitivities, skin breakouts, and beyond.

Even if you are eating healthily or drinking green juice, if your body can't break down and rid itself of unwanted waste and toxins in your food, water, coffee, hygiene and cleaning products, or environment, you become toxic—as I did.

## BECOMING TOXIC FROM MY ENVIRONMENT

I survived mold. Barely.

Before getting sick, I'd heard of people getting sick from mold exposure, but I never thought much about it. Until it happened to me.

Some people can be exposed to mold day in, day out, and be completely fine. Others merely sniff it on a piece of food or clothing and are sent into a toxic tailspin. As you can probably guess, I fell into the latter category. My body could not eliminate it properly.

Mold causes oxidative stress, triggers inflammation, worsens immune function, causes uncomfortable and itchy rashes and hives, sinus congestion, insomnia, brain fog, migraines/headaches from brain inflammation, asthma, and so much more. After living in a mold-infested *new* home for two years, the less mold and fungus I could eliminate from my body, the sicker I became—IBS, SIBO, candida, autoimmune disease, and mast cell activation syndrome. Because I also had a long history of dysbiosis, constipation, poor liver health from my long-term restrictive diets, and MTHFR genetic mutation (poor methylation), I was very susceptible to mold illness.

The straw that broke the camel's back—leading me to suspect mold—came at 3 a.m., flat on my back once more in the ER. A Severe asthma attack—again. The doctor couldn't explain it—again. But something in my head flickered: *Mold?* And that's exactly the answer I pursued next.

The next day, a local mold detective, familiar with mold illness, came to my rental to test the air and other spaces in the home. The findings: Black mold spores growing in the heating, ventilation, and air conditioning unit, as well as a wall that had sustained water damage from flooding earlier that year. I was then diagnosed with mycotoxin illness through a urine test, revealing toxic levels of four different types of molds growing inside. Finding mold was only the beginning, though.

I left everything behind. Everything. I "Marie Kondo-ed" my life. It was as if a fire had happened. I got rid of all my furniture, most of my clothes, and my books. It all made me sick. Not everyone with mycotoxin illness has to rid themselves of *everything*, nor are they as sick as I became. But regardless, if you have mold illness, you must initially remove yourself from the environment that is making you ill.

On the medical side of things, I tried everything from IV ozone therapy to rectal and nasal ozone (for mold in the nasal cavity and parasites/mold in the colon), vitamin IVs to boost the immune system, binders like B charcoal, clay, pectin, and chlorella to get the mold out of me. I also detoxed my body with basic intermittent fasting (12 hours overnight from dinner to breakfast the next morning), celery juice, essential oils, colonics, coffee enemas, an infrared sauna, and more.

What I found that absolutely worked the most for my own detox included:

- Pooping daily (using constipation support as needed);
- Sweating and moving daily (appropriate exercise, fresh air, and heated yoga or sauna);
- Lots of water, color-rich vegetables, and simple meals;
- Baseline gut, immune and liver supplementation including short-chain fatty acids, enzymes, antimicrobial herbs, glutathione, Vitamin C, and binders to support digestion and elimination.

Although it would take a solid two years until I started to feel like a new woman, I healed and quickly discovered that unless we support our elimination pathways, our toxic world is not going anywhere anytime soon.

# OUR TOXIC WORLD

We live in a toxic world. Every day, Americans are exposed to thousands of unseen chemicals and toxins.

A toxin is a poisonous substance made by a living organism (biotoxin).

Of the eighty thousand-plus chemicals currently used in the US, nearly 90 percent of these toxins and chemicals have not been adequately tested for their safety or effects on human health. Moreover, the average American uses 126 unregulated chemicals on their body alone in about nine different personal care products before they leave the house every morning.

To put this in context, Europe has banned over 1,300 chemicals, but the US has only banned about thirty. Chemical guidelines for most hygiene and home cleaning supplies have not been updated since 1938, when a law was passed, giving the FDA almost no authority to regulate these products. Companies are allowed to put nearly any chemical into personal care and learning products sold in the US without any safety testing and without disclosing all the chemicals on labels, including several known carcinogens and endocrine disruptors, like coal tar, talc, formaldehyde, and lead acetate.

Other common toxic chemicals we are exposed to regularly include pesticides sprayed on your broccoli and GMO apples, hydrogenated vegetable oils in your Chinese food takeout, synthetic chemicals lurking in your mattress, artificial sweeteners and food additives, heavy metals in our braces and seafood, and hormones in the chicken on our dinner plates. Beyond hidden chemicals, environmental exposures, including those found in our water supply and biotoxins (like mold), air pollution, radiation, and electromagnetic fields are also of concern.

Although there are many perks about living in modern times—from indoor heating and air conditioning to broccoli from two thousand miles away readily available at our local Whole Foods and rose-blossom-scented body wash—these perks come with their share of repercussions. The world we live in today is starkly different from the environment in which humans were meant to evolve and thrive.

We live indoors, in homes full of chemicals, trapped air, and off-gassing chemicals from paints, upholstery, and furniture. We wash ourselves with chemical-infused cleansers—many contaminated with additional toxic chemicals not listed on the labels. We drink water containing metals and contaminants like lead, fluoride, and chromium, which are not meant to hydrate us. We eat foods sprayed with pesticides or chemicals synthesized in a factory to taste like food. The story goes on.

Unfortunately, with regular and repeat exposure, we humans become easy targets for these toxins to overthrow our natural digestive and eliminatory processes, turning us into bio-accumulators. Over four hundred chemicals have been identified in human tissues and cells, which further decrease the strength of our elimination pathways.

One research study of newborn babies found upwards of 287 chemicals in their umbilical cords alone—180 of those chemicals are known to cause cancer in humans or animals, and 217 are known to be toxic to the brain and nervous system. Another study, this time evaluating urine glyphosate levels in adults, found that human exposure to glyphosate, a chemical widely found in weed killers, has increased by approximately 500 percent since the introduction of genetically modified crops over a 23-year span. The findings sparked an uproar, particularly in the agriculture and food industry, as well as further demand for more research on the long-term side effects of glyphosate (commercial name, Roundup), which is currently the most-used weed killer for use around produce in the US and found in most processed, packaged foods, gluten-containing foods, and restaurant seed oils nationwide.

It's not just what you eat though, but how you eat and the chemicals in our environment as well. Research shows that in your kitchen, using non-stick pans (like Teflon cookware) for just 2-5 minutes can exceed temperatures at which the coating breaks apart and emits toxic particles and gasses linked to hundreds, perhaps thousands, of pet bird deaths and an unknown number of human illnesses each year. Meanwhile, dishwasher and hand soap with triclosan, an aggressive antibacterial agent, can promote the growth of drug-resistant bacteria—even without taking antibiotics. Even if a product says "Green," "Eco," "Hypoallergenic," or "Natural," there are no legal standards for these terms, and many of these products contain potent allergens, such as formaldehyde-releasing preservatives or fragrances.

As mentioned earlier in this book, it is suspected that 50 percent of homes and buildings in the US have water damage and mold toxicity. Even in buildings without water damage, mold and other fungi and bacterium can develop when indoor humidity levels reach around 50-60 percent. For this reason, many signs and symptoms of mycotoxin exposure fly under the radar, believed to be the norm—such as sinus congestion attributed to allergies, morning stiffness, or frequent loose stool. Still, others struggle with co-morbidities associated with mold exposure, like autoimmune disease, weight gain/loss, hormone imbalances, or skin conditions that will not heal, no matter the treatments sought.

Although toxins are inevitable, and we cannot live in bubbles to escape them, we *do* have the ability to support our detox pathways by at least offsetting some of these contaminants by avoiding them when we can and integrating simple detox practices into our daily lives.

## HOW TO DETOX SMART

Have you ever washed greasy dishes without hot water or dish soap? The dishes don't get clean, do they? When toxic metals and chemical food additives get inside your body, it takes a strong cleanser to scrub your body clean from the inside out.

Although you may think about juice cleanses, fasting, coffee enemas, and sweat lodge retreats when you hear the word "detox," detoxing does not have to be extreme and is something your body can do naturally, daily.

In fact, extremes, such as fasting, can have the opposite effects—releasing more toxins into the body or inhibiting the body from detoxing due to a lack of nutrients and liver-supportive herbs, foods, and/or helpful supplements. In particular, cleansing requires antioxidants (found in vegetables) and proteins, especially bone broths, wild-caught fish, and organic meats (like skin-on pastured chicken thighs, grass-fed, grass-finished beef, and organ meats) in order to stimulate liver detox. Without enough nutrients for your liver, detoxification stalls.

A *smart* (not crazy restrictive) detox simply entails intentionally supporting and strengthening your eight cleansing channels through cleansing foods, lifestyle factors, and smart supplementation (no Grapefruit Diet required).

The key to detoxing is making conscious choices on a daily basis that *reduce* toxin exposure and allow your channels to "flow."

One of the simplest ways to do this is by gradually replacing toxic commercial products (cleaning, hygiene, beauty supplies) and materials (cooking supplies, utensils, bedding, furniture, etc.) in your home with non-toxic versions. You don't have to break the bank overnight, but as you run out of soaps, face washes, and mascara, begin changing out the brands you use. The Environmental Working Group's website (EWG.org) has several very helpful guides for choosing the best toxic-free products, air purifiers, water filters, and foods for a toxin-free home.

On the food front, avoiding toxins is a no-brainer, including pesticides, fertilizers, and mycotoxin-laden foods, along with hormone and antibiotic-enriched "natural" meats (marketing, people). Eat as local and organic as possible—we eat what our animals eat and are given, along with the chemicals sprayed on our apples, spinach, and even gluten-free rice cakes. This explains why many people may go on a gluten-free diet and eat all the gluten-free goodies yet continue to feel worse, not better. Similarly, gluten-containing foods, like bread, cereals, and pasta, have over a 90 percent likelihood of mycotoxin contamination—toxic mold spores, glyphosate contamination, or both, along with other pesticides.

Is it really gluten intolerance or something else in gluten making many of us sick and disrupting our gut?

Additionally, you can support your detox pathways by taking proactive steps to detox daily—*especially* making sure you are sweating and having regular bowel movements to clear waste. If you are *not* pooping daily, then Houston, we have a problem!

How can you naturally support healthy poo? On top of boosting stomach acid and enzyme production with digestive bitters, enzymes, and foods (Superpower 3), other helpful poo supports may include magnesium citrate (taken before bed), high-dose buffered Vitamin C powder (1000 mg taken 2-3 times per day), ginger and peppermint tea, eating vegetables cooked, pureed, or sauteed, low-FODMAP foods, activated charcoal or *Saccharomyces boulardii* (for loose stools), and coffee enemas (for chronic constipation).

## WHAT ABOUT PARASITES?

All people have microscopic parasites living inside them, just like all people have bacteria, viruses, and germs living inside them at all times.

In medical terms, a parasite is an organism that lives on or in a host organism and gets its food from or at the expense of its host. Parasites feed on the nutrients that are meant for us.

Parasites or "protozoa" are a normal part of life. In fact, over 3,200 species of parasites are found everywhere in our environment—in the air we breathe, the water we drink, and the foods we eat. Consequently, these parasites easily make their way into our own GI tracts as well, where they live alongside a host of other good and bad bacteria and fungi.

Many people go their whole lives without knowing they have parasites in them. Many are harmless to the human body if you have a strong immune system, plenty of healthy gut bacteria, and good detoxification systems working for you. However, if your immune system, gut health, and/or detox pathways are down (from stress and inflammation), then you are more likely to become the perfect "host" for a parasite to take over and cause inflammation.

Additionally, we can come into contact with *new* parasites in food, water, air, soil, hospitals, foreign country travel, etc., and instantly become susceptible to developing a parasitic infection if our immune defenses are "unarmed." For example, food poisoning from Chinese takeout, drinking bad water in Mexico, getting bitten by a tick or flea, or swimming in a fresh body of water and then becoming ill are all examples of how new parasites living outside of us can hijack our health.

Parasites are the X-factor that can be kept undercover and harmless if our body is generally healthy and on it's A-game, but in the blink of an eye, parasites can take our health south fast if our immune defenses, gut bacteria, and/or detox system are "unarmed."

## TESTING FOR PARASITES

So, how do you know if you have parasites and if you should treat them?

Testing for parasites is tricky—primarily because parasites LOVE to hide out in nooks, crannies, and biofilm. Biofilm is sort of like dental plaque on your teeth—a thick protective sticky goo composed of bacteria and fungi that form a steel-like armor casing around certain parasites and other bacteria and fungi in order to protect them and keep them alive in your body.

A good first place to start with "testing" is to assess if you have any parasite-infection-related symptoms.

*Parasite Infection Symptoms:*

- GI symptoms (constipation, diarrhea, IBS, bloating, nausea);
- Unintended weight loss or weight gain;
- A slow or fast metabolism;
- Fatigue (despite sleeping);
- Cravings for sugar/sweets/carbs/snacks;
- Low iron, low ferritin, low Vitamin B12 and/or anemia of chronic disease;
- Shortness of breath/air hunger;

- Anxiety or depression;
- Brain fog/difficulty concentrating;
- Hormone imbalances (irregular periods, horrible PMS, hot flashes, breast tenderness);
- Autoimmune flares;
- Mast cell activation syndrome flares[2];
- Not "healing" (despite eating well, exercising, and drinking water).

The symptoms of parasite infection can be similar to symptoms of other underlying conditions as well, such as mold illness, Lyme disease, SIBO, or simply impaired gut function, and often are not isolated, meaning other conditions may be at play.

Beyond parasite infection symptoms, lab testing may be helpful, although lab testing frequently still misses parasites because, again, the critters like to hide.

## PARASITE CLEANSE

With or without formal testing, a gentle, "broad spectrum" parasite cleanse may be worth considering *after* you've dialed your foundational Superpowers into place. However, be warned: There are tons of misguided parasite cleanse tips and tricks out there on the internet—many that can lead to ill parasite cleanse side effects if you are unaware of how to properly cleanse.

Any good parasite cleanse will *not* jump into treating or "cleansing" out the parasite right away with harsh antimicrobial herbs or antibiotics without first preparing your body to do so; otherwise, you may run into cleanse side effects or "die off reactions"—also known as "Herx" reactions.

Once the foundations are in place, you can move into detoxing parasites or other toxins more directly while keeping up your foundational supports. You may integrate:

**More binder support**—to "mop up" toxins. I use a blend of Zeolite, Chlorella, BioActive Carbon, Modified Citrus Pectin, and occasionally activated charcoal or bentonite clay, although I find those two to be a bit more constipating if you are prone to constipation.

2 https://www.ncbi.nlm.nih.gov/pmc/articles/PMC5382204/

**Anti-parasitic, anti-bacterial, and anti-fungal herbs:**

- Oregano leaf;
- Cat's claw;
- Hydrastis (goldenseal);
- Coptis;
- Garlic or allicin;
- Caprylic acid;
- Bearberry;
- Berberis (barberry);
- Black Walnut;
- Berberine HCL.
- Mimosa Pudica Seed: Seeds that gently but effectively help pull parasites out of your system;
- Cistus tea or cistus tea extract: 1-3 cups per day, as tolerated, to disrupt biofilm.

During your cleanse, continue to nourish your body—not deprive it—with real nutrient-dense foods—optimal liver function requires amino acids, antioxidants, hydration, and fatty acids to work effectively.

Generally, most parasite cleanses will last about thirty days unless severe fungal and bacterial overgrowth are also at play. It is highly advised you work with a knowledgeable clinician or healthcare practitioner familiar with parasite cleanses to avoid damage to your gut.

# MINDSET CONSTIPATION

Speaking of poo, mindset constipation is another trigger of poor detox that is worth considering.

Mindset constipation is a phenomenon describing how stress (such as feeling overwhelmed, stretching yourself too thin, and negative thinking) results in symptoms such as constipation and bloating, no matter how few FODMAPs you eat or Smooth Move tea you drink.

## *WHAT ARE YOU FEEDING YOUR MIND?*

We are what we eat, and we are what we think.

Eat potato chips, soda, and Ben & Jerry's every day, and chances are your gut microbiome will feel like potato chips, soda, and Ben & Jerry's, resulting in low energy, blood sugar imbalances, and insatiable cravings. Eat healing herbs and broth, fresh fruits and veggies, and hydrating water every day, and chances are your gut microbiome will feel like it—full of energy, vibrancy, and cleansed.

The same thing goes for what you feed your mind. YouTube cat videos, Netflix, social media scrolling, negative political news feeds, gossip, trashy reality TV shows, and negative conversations (with yourself and others) produce one type of mindset. Growth mindset-type books, podcasts, conversations, positive experiences, mantras, and devotionals produce another.

Did you know that you have upwards of 50,000-80,000 thoughts in a given day? Of these thoughts, more than 80 percent are negative, and 90 percent are repeat thoughts you have had before. It's important to realize that your thoughts—the ones going through your head 24/7—are not always true. Rather, many of our thoughts are downloads—things we've been told at one time or believed at one time to be true, and they've stuck with us.

For example, "I will never get married," "I'll never get a raise," "No one likes me," or "I will always struggle with X" can be toxic thoughts that we never second guess because we have believed them for far too long—even if they are not true.

Over time, if we stay stuck in this negative-thinking loop, we weigh ourselves down—mindset constipation.

We are not only what we eat; we are also what eats us.

## FILLS AND DRAINS

The concept of fills and drains describes the activities, thoughts, habits, and tasks we let into our lives—and if they are energizing (filling) or energy-depriving (draining) for our well-being.

Like a 24-ounce cup that can only hold 24 ounces of water, we all only get 24 hours in a day, and we get to choose what fills or drains that cup.

When our cup is full but just right (not too full), we experience more inner peace and less mindset constipation. When our cup is way too full, it overflows, consequently draining that cup, and our Brain-Gut Connection feels it.

# GUT LOVE HABIT 7: DETOX DAILY

*Sweat. Flush. Poo.* Integrate at least *one* daily detox practice to support your elimination pathways (it can be the same one if you like or several).

## *SWEAT:*

Sweat daily (beyond just a workout)—sauna sessions, steamy hot showers, detox baths, heated yoga.

## *FLUSH:*

Drink celery juice on an empty stomach (after 16-20 oz water). Try dry brushing, back lying with your legs up a wall while deep breathing, or rebounding.

## *POO:*

First thing in the morning, give yourself at least 5-10 minutes to release. Sit upright on the loo, and throughout the day, for better stool elimination since slouching prevents food peristalsis (movement), decreases stomach acid, and inhibits full elimination. If you *still* struggle to poo, try the Golden Poo hacks:

## *CONSTIPATION HACKS:*

- Drink enough water *with* minerals—a pinch of sea salt will do a couple of times per day;
- Sip Smooth Move tea before bed;
- Supplement with 1-2 droppers of digestive bitters with meals;
- Add magnesium citrate and/or buffered Vitamin C to your supplement routine;
- Coffee enema;
- Drink 4-8 oz of prune juice plus one tablespoon of extra virgin olive oil or grass-fed butter. Drink it for a quick elimination;
- Take high dose digestive enzymes with meals (2-4 capsules) and/or a "gut love shot" (1-2 tbsp of apple cider vinegar in 4-8 oz of water);
- Eat food for breakfast (vs. fasting or drinking a smoothie) and/or add resistant starch or soluble fiber with dinner to support a morning stool.

## *LOOSE STOOL HACKS:*

- Chlorella tablets or activated charcoal;
- Take *Saccharomyces boulardii*;
- Include carob powder in your diet or make your own homemade carob "coffee";
- Consider addressing SIBO with a practitioner using an antimicrobial herbal protocol (once diet and lifestyle changes have been made).

## *EXPERIMENT 1: SIMPLE SWAPS:*

Gradually replace toxic versions of your hygiene, cleaning, cooking, home, and beauty products with non-toxic versions. As you run out of fluoride-rich toothpaste, opt for a fluoride-free version. Ditch the plastic water bottles in favor of glass or stainless steel drinking containers. Shop around for a non-toxic mattress—especially if you're due for an upgrade. Toss the talc-rich blush for a non-toxic cream blush.

## *EXPERIMENT 2: QUICK GALLBLADDER AND LIVER FLUSH:*

Push a "reset" button for your liver and gallbladder: Perform a quick liver-gallbladder "flush."

**Day 1:**
Eat a lower-fat diet on the day of the liver flush. Starting at 6 p.m., follow the steps below:

6:00 p.m. – stop eating or drinking.
8:00 p.m. – mix and drink the following to have a bowel movement in 1-2 hours:

- 8 oz. pure apple juice;
- 1 tablespoon Epsom Salt.

10:00 p.m.– mix and drink the following:

- 4 oz. red grapefruit juice from one grapefruit or lemon juice;
- 4 oz. olive oil;
- 4 oz. classic coke.

After drinking the juice, coke, and olive oil mixture, immediately lay down on your right side and bring your right leg up near your chest for about 45 minutes. Try to sleep on the right side, close to the fetal position, for the rest of the night.

**Day 2**

Upon waking, repeat the apple juice and Epsom Salt drink to encourage another bowel movement.

Optional: Do one coffee enema during the day.

Notes:

If you do not have a bowel movement within 1-2 hours of taking the first apple juice and Epsom Salt drink, continue with the rest of the flush instructions. On your next attempt at a flush, stop eating at 4:00 p.m. and drink the apple juice and Epsom Salt drink at 6:00 p.m. and again at 8:00 p.m. and continue with the rest of the flush as above. Conversely, if you have a very short transit time, consume less Epsom Salt and drink just enough of it to give you a good bowel movement before drinking the juice, coke, and olive oil mixture.

The coke may be omitted, but certain ingredients specific to coke are helpful in reducing nausea and softening toxic matter. The benefit of flush will likely outweigh the negative effects of the coke.

# CHAPTER 18:
# SUPERPOWER 8: CONNECTION

You and your gut bugs were not made to be alone.

All humans are innately wired to thrive in tribes—doing life with other people. Long before the University of Texas Longhorn fans and the Backstreet Boys teen groupies, group camaraderie was a way for our ancestors to avoid predation, get help finding food, and raise offspring. Connecting with others ensured survival.

Today, our versions of tribes include that recreational softball league, your office co-workers, your family and closest friends, a Bible study group or the members of your book club, a running group you belong to, a basketball team or cheer squad, a Weight Watchers or Whole30 group program, or a political group—mutual connections. Your *need* for tribe is the reason social media is addicting. It is why research shows that there is strength in numbers—armies overthrow empires, "pay it forward" movements spread, and health goals are achieved through group support instead of going it alone.

Newsflash: You are a human *being*. Not a human *doing*. Sometimes we forget this. In fact, eight in ten Americans report being stressed out or exhausted on a regular basis. From long to-do lists to constant pings and messages on our phones, back-to-back meetings or appointments, early wake-ups, and pulling late-nighters, we are constantly "doing" rather than being a "human being."

In the midst of all this running around, not only are we more stressed, but we are also more disconnected, despite being the most connected culture via technology than any other generation in human history.

Mental illness—including anxiety and depression—is at an all-time high, with one in five people struggling with a progressed stage of these two disorders at any point in time. In 2019, Blue Cross Blue Shield released an alarming report revealing that millennials (born 1980-1996) are the "unhealthiest generation" of all time, with the highest rates of chronic illness than any generation before—especially experiencing anxiety and depression from rising debt, substance abuse, loneliness, and lack of meaningful relationships. Another nationwide survey of over twenty thousand Americans found that more than 50 percent of respondents often felt alone and like they have no one they call a close friend; the survey also revealed Gen Z as the loneliest generation in human history, with nearly 70 percent believing they feel like "no one really knows them well."

## UNDERSTANDING THE GUT-SOCIAL CONNECTION

Supportive social relationships and strong connections can tremendously shape your gut microbiota by boosting oxytocin, the feel-good "love hormone." Feelings of confidence, happiness, and that general "glow" of health radiate from the brain to the gut, cultivating a hospitable environment.

Our microbes *also* shape our social skills and social personalities. To understand this connection better, researchers looked at the role of the gut microbiome in subjects with autism spectrum disorder (ASD)—a neurodevelopmental disorder characterized by impaired social skills. Since gut issues (like IBS, gluten intolerance, and gas) are common in people with autism, researchers wondered if an impaired gut microbiome also contributes to the manifestation of autism-associated symptoms, such as poor social cues and slowed social and behavioral development. Sure enough, when researchers evaluated the gut bacteria in ASD subjects, it was distinctly different from those of healthy subjects. Then, in three separate trials, when they supported ASD subjects with probiotics—specifically *Lactobacillus reuteri*—their social skills normalized, almost completely improving abnormalities in sociability and enhancing social connections, both in autistic and healthy subjects. The social bacteria sends signals via intestinal neurons, mediating inflammatory effects of gut, hormone, immune, and dietary sensory signals on brain activity. *Lactobacillus reuteri* also promotes oxytocin expression—another win for the "bonding" hormone that makes us want to connect.

Gut microbes are also great matchmakers—helping us attract our friends, partners, and soul mates. We subconsciously determine who we like based on the scent and immune systems of others' gut microbes. One study asked women to rate the attractiveness of a potential partner by smelling their dirty t-shirts. The women did not agree on which smells were the most attractive. Instead, they most often preferred the t-shirt of the man that had the most complimentary immune system that would broaden their offspring's spectrum of immunity. The strange thing is that the immune genes and resulting sweat don't have much of a smell. Instead, a person's body odor comes from the specific microbes that consume their sweat, skin cells, and oils. So the women smelling the dirty t-shirts were not smelling the men's immune system genes directly, but they could sense the small differences that the immune system had, depending on the type of microbes that grew.

And have you ever heard the saying, "we are a sum of the five people closest to us?" Well, we tend to share microbes with the people closest to us. Researchers can tell who we are related to just by sequencing our gut bacteria alone; microbial communities in each home are easily distinguished from each other. Our microbes are also passed horizontally, from peer to peer. Although we get our first microbes from our moms, these are eventually overwhelmed by those we pick up from friends within a matter of months. This is also why "birds of a feather flock together." Fit people hang with other fit people. Smokers smoke together. Drinkers drink together. Bitcoiners bitcoin together.

This perhaps explains why research in humans reveals copious benefits from relationships on our total health. Strong social connections have been shown to increase longevity by 50 percent, strengthen your immune system, and help you recover from disease faster. Lack of social connection, on the other hand, is a greater detriment to health than obesity, smoking, and high blood pressure. The biomes of older adults living in institutions, such as skilled nursing facilities versus neighborhood and retirement communities, vary significantly, with less diversity and bacteria overall among those living in an institution.

People living in the Blue Zones are a perfect example of this. The Blue Zones are coined "the five healthiest communities in the world," where the people live the longest and are the happiest, including the Barbagia region of

Sardinia in Italy, Ikaria in Greece, Okinawa in Japan, the Nicoya Peninsula in Costa Rica, and Loma Linda, California. People in these Blue Zones regions don't just live longer; they live better. Besides having a large number of centenarians, people in these areas remain active into their 80s and 90s and, for the most part, do not suffer from the chronic diseases common in most parts of the industrialized world. Initially, when researchers set out to uncover why exactly people in the Blue Zones are healthier and happier, they looked first to DNA and geography (location), with inconclusive evidence. After a little more digging, they soon discovered the following "Power 9" reasons for the unique health of the inhabitants of Blue Zones.

1. Moving naturally throughout the day;
2. Having and cultivating a strong sense of purpose;
3. Downshifting every day to relieve stress;
4. Following the 80 percent rule: Stop eating when 80 percent full;
5. Making veggies and fruit the center of their diet;
6. Enjoying wine and alcohol moderately with friends and/or food;
7. Belonging to faith-based communities or other organizations;
8. Putting loved ones first, having close friends and strong family connections;
9. Cultivating close friends and strong social networks.

Notice that four of these Power 9 reasons have *nothing* to do with diet, supplements, or exercise; people and a sense of connection.

Researchers took their observations a step further, evaluating why the communities full of healthy aging seniors (ages 70-90), coined "SuperAgers," had distinctive brain features, including thicker cortexes, a resistance to age-related atrophy, and a larger left anterior cingulate (a part of the brain important to attention and working memory). They asked 31 SuperAgers and 19 cognitively "normal" older adults to fill out a 42-item questionnaire about their psychological well-being. The SuperAgers stood out in one area: The degree to which they reported having satisfying, warm, trusting relationships.

## SPARK JOY

What would you spend your time doing if you had complete financial abundance to do anything? What gets your heart or energy pumping? What energizes you? What brings purpose to your days—are you living your purpose?

Aside from human connection, connection to things that "Spark Joy" in our lives *and our* purpose is a superpower rarely discussed in health circles.

"Sparking Joy" is all about intentionally creating or finding a *little* bit of joy, or sense of calm and peace, in your daily life— an activity, an experience, an observation—like a really cool conversation with a new friend or the grocery store clerk, your morning routine, or that cup of coffee that you savor.

I originally developed the Spark Joy concept after reading a book by organization expert Marie Kando called *The Life Changing Magic of Tidying Up*. In her book, Marie teaches readers how to declutter their lives by going through their clutter, room by room, and asking themselves one question when trying to decide whether to throw something away or keep it: "Does it Spark Joy?" If you don't feel joy about an item, get rid of it. As a result, you're free from that four-sizes-too-small little black dress bought half off at TJ Maxx three years ago and the forty Beanie Babies collecting dust in a box under your bed. You are free from things weighing you down.

While the practice is game-changing for your closet, I've found "Sparking Joy" to be even more game-changing for healing—both for myself and my patients like Kelly.

Kelly, 33, couldn't lose those last 10 pounds or bloating or constipation no matter what she tried. On top of that, she couldn't sleep, getting only around 4 hours per night. Her hair was also falling out, her skin was breaking out, and she just didn't "feel like herself," despite eating clean, taking supplements, and doing deep breathing to help. Early on in her treatment, I prescribed: "Make a list of five to ten things that bring you joy and that you love to do—big or small. Drinking your morning cup of coffee at your favorite coffee shop to time in the day to write or paint, hip-hop dance, walking at Town Lake. Anything."

A week later, Kelly had a list of almost sixty things that sparked joy.

The challenge: "Incorporate at least *one* Spark Joy into your life each day and get connected to something—even just *one* thing that is a reflection of your 'Spark Joy' list. See how it changes the trajectory of how you feel physically and mentally."

Four weeks later, the bloating and constipation were gone, and Kelly was sleeping eight hours through the night. The scale was finally budging.

Crucially, there was no further change in diet or exercise at all. Kelly flipped the script by seeing the glass of her life as half full versus half empty and choosing to be at Cause vs. Effect.

People with a higher sense of purpose in their days have almost 50 percent greater health and mental-emotional outcomes than those who wander aimlessly.

Get connected. Spark Joy.

*Tip: Feeling purposeless?*
*One of my absolute favorite books is The Purpose Driven Life by Rick Warren. Check it out.*

## GUT LOVE HABIT #8: CONNECT

Pay it forward to boost your gut bugs. Intentionally conduct an experiment (or two or five) to perform a random act of kindness for someone else. Bake (gluten-free) cookies for a friend or neighbor, call an old friend to let them know you're thinking of them, smile at someone and compliment them, and surprise your letter carrier with a letter to them in the mailbox. Go out of your way. In turn, you do your body and gut some good.

### *GUT RESET EXPERIMENT: BUILD YOUR TRIBE*

Build your "tribe." Take the extra step to connect or cultivate community in at least one area of your life:

- Join a community service organization;
- Connect with a fitness community or two—yoga studio, gym, fitness classes;
- Connect with a spiritual community;
- Try local meet-ups around hobbies that interest you—hiking, cycling, photography, etc.;
- Join business-related groups and organizations;
- Attend support groups;
- Support groups around like-minded goals in your life;

- Make a hang-out date with an old friend, a new friend, a co-worker, or someone in your community you have been meaning to get to know;
- Go the extra mile and plan or host a meet-up with several friends, such as a dinner night at your house, a board game night, a pickup soccer game or other event.

## THE BOTTOM LINE

You (and your gut bugs) were not meant to be alone. Quality relationships and communities are another powerful, natural de-stressor and gut microbial booster, and a healthy, happy gut is a powerful social network and stress-resilience booster.

## GUT CHECK POINT

Your body has the power to heal itself; all you have to do is support it. There is no faster or more effective way to reduce inflammation and jump-start healing than by "weeding and seeding"; weeding out the toxins and stressful habits dragging you down and seeding your Eight Gut Love Superpowers for a Total Gut Reset.

A quick reminder: Your Eight Superpowers are:

1. Breath
2. Hydration
3. Digestion
4. Nutrients
5. Rest
6. Movement
7. Detox
8. Connection

In clinical practice, I've seen 90 percent of my clients transform their health by optimizing these Superpowers alone. When in doubt about how to heal, first and foremost, always come back to your baseline.

## WHAT ABOUT PROTOCOLS, DIETS, AND SUPPLEMENTS?

Supplements and specific therapeutic diets and protocols (like the "SIBO protocol" or "mold protocol") are often part of a Total Gut Reset once your Gut Love Superpowers are established. I wish I could cover every single possible condition and symptom out there, along with specific protocols and treatments that are effective. However, if I gave you a one-size-fits-all approach, we would be here for a very long time. This is where customization and working with a skilled functional medicine clinician or joining a program like the Total Gut Reset comes into play. To steer you in the right direction, I've included some general but effective recommendations on the best foods and supplements for each Gut Type in the *Resources: Eat and Supplement for Your Gut Type* section at the back of this book.

## GUT LOVE RITUALS

It would be remiss of me to fall into the trap of giving you all of this information without providing a practical framework to follow that would allow you to take real steps in the right direction.

Again, there is detailed information contained within the Resources section of this book, but the Three Gut Love Rituals below, if performed daily, will help you build the right habits and routines that will get you moving in the right direction.

### *BREAKFAST*

- Hydrate: Drink 8 to 16 oz warm lemon water and a pinch of sea salt. Optional: 8 ounces fresh celery juice.
- Protein Up: Power up with protein in your morning meal (at least 20 grams).
- Get Your Mind Right: Journal your affirmations, top 1 to 3 intentions or "to dos" for the day, and your "breath prayers."

## DURING THE DAY

- Boost Your Energy: Instead of coffee or sugar, reach for an "energizing" greens powder, bone broth, cacao, or tea. Pair with a little protein or healthy fat if a snack craving strikes.
- Just Breathe: Inhale essential oils, like energizing peppermint, on your pulse points and under your nostrils, close your eyes, and "just breathe" for 1 to 2 minutes.
- Move It, Move It: Move your body in some way at some point (or two) during the day every day, whether you have 7 minutes or 60. Some people love morning workouts. Others do better with a mid-day or post-work movement block, or intermixed "recess" breaks throughout the day. Walking, bodyweight movements and mobility never go out of style (especially if there's a great music playlist involved).

## BED

- Tea Time: Drink tea or cacao "hot chocolate" for a gut love treat.
- Candle Down: Get your body prepped for quality R&R in the evening. Turn bright and overhead lights off and use lamps, candles, and/or red, blue-blocking glasses. Take a hot shower or bath, hit a sauna session, warming yoga flow, then sleep in a pitch-black cooled room, ideally at 68 degrees or below.
- Get Your Mind Right: Journal your top 1 to 3 "cool things" or "gratitudes" from the day; log any "to dos" you may have for tomorrow, and bullet journal your "breath prayers."

## REFERENCES


1. Voucher Cloud. 2019. How Many Productive Hours in a Work Day? Just 2 Hours, 23 Minutes. https://www.vouchercloud.com/blog/office-worker-productivity/
2. Fluoride Action Network. 2019. http://fluoridealert.org/content/bfs-2012/
3. Kanduti, D., Sterbenk, P., & Artnik, B. 2016. FLUORIDE: A REVIEW OF USE AND EFFECTS ON HEALTH. *Materia socio-medica, 28*(2), 133–137. doi:10.5455/msm.2016.28.133-137
4. NRDC. 2019. The Truth About Tap. https://www.nrdc.org/stories/truth-about-tap

5. David, L. A., Maurice, C. F., Carmody, R. N., Gootenberg, D. B., Button, J. E., Wolfe, B. E., ... Turnbaugh, P. J. (2014). Diet rapidly and reproducibly alters the human gut microbiome. *Nature, 505*(7484), 559–563. doi:10.1038/nature12820

6. Food Information Council. 2019. 2019 Food & Health Survey. https://foodinsight.org/wp-content/uploads/2019/05/IFIC-Foundation-2019-Food-and-Health-Report-FINAL.pdf

7. Govender, M., Choonara, Y. E., Kumar, P., du Toit, L. C., van Vuuren, S., & Pillay, V. (2013). A review of the advancements in probiotic delivery: Conventional vs. non-conventional formulations for intestinal flora supplementation. *AAPS PharmSciTech, 15*(1), 29–43. doi:10.1208/s12249-013-0027-1

8. Satish S. C. Rao, Abdul Rehman, Siegfried Yu, Nicole Martinez de Andino. Brain fogginess, gas and bloating: a link between SIBO, probiotics and metabolic acidosis. *Clinical and Translational Gastroenterology*, 2018; 9 (6) DOI: 10.1038/s41424-018-0030-7

9. Scourboutakos, M. J., Franco-Arellano, B., Murphy, S. A., Norsen, S., Comelli, E. M., & L'Abbé, M. R. (2017). Mismatch between Probiotic Benefits in Trials versus Food Products. *Nutrients, 9*(4), 400. doi:10.3390/nu9040400

10. Capela, P. & Hay, T.K.C. & Shah, Nagendra. (2006). Effect of cryoprotectants, prebiotics and microencapsulation on survival of probiotic organisms in yogurt and freeze-dried yogurt. Food Research International. 39. 203-211. 10.1016/j.foodres.2005.07.007.

11. Environmental Working Group. 2019. Skin Deep Database. https://www.ewg.org/skindeep/

12. Rea, W. 1996. Chemical Sensitivity: Tools, Diagnosis and Method of Treatment, Volume 4.

13. Environmental Working Group. 2005. Body Burden: The Pollution in Newborns. https://www.ewg.org/research/body-burden-pollution-newborns

14. Gillezeau, C., van Gerwen, M., Shaffer, R. M., Rana, I., Zhang, L., Sheppard, L., & Taioli, E. (2019). The evidence of human exposure to glyphosate: a review. *Environmental health : a global access science source, 18*(1), 2. doi:10.1186/s12940-018-0435-5

15. Environmental Working Group. 2003. Canaries in the Kitchen. https://www.ewg.org/research/canaries-kitchen

16. Berkeley Lab. 2009. Indoor Air Quality: Scientific Findings Resource Bank. https://iaqscience.lbl.gov/dampness-prevalence

17. Reponen, T., Levin, L., Zheng, S., Vesper, S., Ryan, P., Grinshpun, S. A., & LeMasters, G. (2013). Family and home characteristics correlate with mold in homes. *Environmental research, 124*, 67–70. doi:10.1016/j.envres.2013.04.003

18. Spengler J, Neas L, Nakai S, Dockery D, Speizer F, Ware J, Raizenne M. Respiratory symptoms and housing characteristics. Indoor Air. 1994;4:72–82.

19. Stephen J. Carter, Gary R. Hunter, J. Walker Blackston, Nianjun Liu, Elliot J. Lefkowitz, William J. Van Der Pol, Casey D. Morrow, Jesseca A. Paulsen, Laura Q. Rogers. Gut microbiota diversity associates with cardiorespiratory fitness in post-primary treatment breast cancer survivors. *Experimental Physiology*, 2019; DOI: 10.1113/EP087404

20. Allen, Jacob & Mailing, Lucy & Niemiro, Grace & Moore, Rachel & Cook, Mark & White, Bryan & Holscher, Hannah & Woods, Jeffrey. (2017). Exercise Alters Gut Microbiota Composition and Function in Lean and Obese Humans. Medicine & Science in Sports & Exercise. 50. 1. 10.1249/MSS.0000000000001495.

21. Lambert, J. E. *et al.* Exercise training modifies gut microbiota in normal and diabetic mice. *Appl. Physiol. Nutr. Metab.* 40, 749–752 (2015).

22. Campbell, S. C. *et al.* The Effect of Diet and Exercise on Intestinal Integrity and Microbial Diversity in Mice. *PloS One* 11, e0150502 (2016).

23. Lamprecht, M., Bogner, S., Schippinger, G., Steinbauer, K., Fankhauser, F., Hallstroem, S., ... Greilberger, J. F. (2012). Probiotic supplementation affects markers of intestinal barrier, oxidation, and inflammation in trained men; a randomized, double-blinded, placebo-controlled trial. *Journal of the International Society of Sports Nutrition, 9*(1), 45. doi:10.1186/1550-2783-9-45

24. Jeukendrup AE, Vet-Joop K, Sturk A, *et al.* Relationship between gastro-intestinal complaints and endotoxaemia, cytokine release and the acute-phase reaction during and after a long-distance triathlon in highly trained men. Clin Sci (Lond) 2000;98:47 55. doi: 10.1042/cs0980047.

25. Liew, W. P., & Mohd-Redzwan, S. (2018). Mycotoxin: Its Impact on Gut Health and Microbiota. *Frontiers in cellular and infection microbiology, 8,* 60. https://doi.org/10.3389/fcimb.2018.00060

26. Crabtree, D.P.E., Herrera, B.J. & Kang, S. The response of human bacteria to static magnetic field and radiofrequency electromagnetic field. *J Microbiol.* **55**, 809–815 (2017) doi:10.1007/s12275-017-7208-7

27. Blachier, François & Beaumont, Martin & Portune, Kevin & Steuer, Nils & Lan, Annaïg & Audebert, Marc & Khodorova, Nadezda & Andriamihaja, Mireille & Airinei, Gheorghe & Benamouzig, Robert & Davila, Anne-Marie & Armand, Lucie & Rampelli, Simone & Brigidi, Patrizia & Tomé, Daniel & Claus, Sandrine & Sanz, Yolanda. (2018). High-protein diets for weight management: Interactions with the intestinal microbiota and consequences for gut health. A position paper by the My New Gut study group. Clinical Nutrition. 38. 10.1016/j.clnu.2018.09.016.

28. Madsen, L., Myrmel, L. S., Fjære, E., Liaset, B., & Kristiansen, K. (2017). Links between Dietary Protein Sources, the Gut Microbiota, and Obesity. *Frontiers in physiology, 8,* 1047. doi:10.3389/fphys.2017.01047

29. Allaband, C., McDonald, D., Vázquez-Baeza, Y., Minich, J. J., Tripathi, A., Brenner, D. A., ... Knight, R. (2019). Microbiome 101: Studying, Analyzing, and Interpreting Gut Microbiome Data for Clinicians. *Clinical gastroenterology and hepatology : the official clinical practice journal of the American Gastroenterological Association, 17*(2), 218–230. doi:10.1016/j.cgh.2018.09.017

30. David, L. A., Maurice, C. F., Carmody, R. N., Gootenberg, D. B., Button, J. E., Wolfe, B. E., ... Turnbaugh, P. J. (2014). Diet rapidly and reproducibly alters the human gut microbiome. *Nature, 505*(7484), 559–563. doi:10.1038/nature12820

31. Widdowson, E. & Oftedal, Olav & Speth, John D & Foley, R. & Soest, P.. (1991). Protein Selection and Avoidance Strategies of Contemporary and Ancestral Foragers: Unresolved Issues: Discussion. Royal Society of London Philosophical Transactions Series B. 334. 10.1098/rstb.1991.0115.

32. Gardner CD, Trepanowski JF, Del Gobbo LC, *et al.* Effect of Low-Fat vs Low-Carbohydrate Diet on 12-Month Weight Loss in Overweight Adults and the Association With Genotype Pattern or Insulin Secretion: The DIETFITS Randomized Clinical Trial. *JAMA.* 2018;319(7):667–679. doi:https://doi.org/10.1001/jama.2018.0245

33. Wan, Yi & Wang, Fenglei & Yuan, Jihong & Li, Jie & Jiang, Dandan & Zhang, Jingjing & Li, Hao & Wang, Ruoyi & Tang, Jun & Huang, Tao & Zheng, Ju-Sheng & Sinclair, Andrew & Mann, Jim. (2019). Effects of dietary fat on gut microbiota and faecal metabolites, and their relationship with cardiometabolic risk factors: A 6-month randomised controlled-feeding trial. Gut. 68. gutjnl-2018. 10.1136/gutjnl-2018-317609.

34. Paoli, A., Mancin, L., Bianco, A., Thomas, E., Mota, J. F., & Piccini, F. (2019). Ketogenic Diet and Microbiota: Friends or Enemies?. *Genes, 10*(7), 534. doi:10.3390/genes10070534

35. Xie, G., Zhou, Q., Qiu, C. Z., Dai, W. K., Wang, H. P., Li, Y H., ... Wang, W. J. (2017). Ketogenic diet poses a significant effect on imbalanced gut microbiota in infants with refractory epilepsy. *World journal of gastroenterology, 23*(33), 6164–6171. doi:10.3748/wjg.v23.i33.6164

36. Leah M. Kalm, Richard D. Semba, They Starved So That Others Be Better Fed: Remembering Ancel Keys and the Minnesota Experiment, *The Journal of Nutrition*, Volume 135, Issue 6, June 2005, Pages 1347–1352, https://doi.org/10.1093/jn/135.6.1347

37. Aird, Tom & Davies, Robert & Carson, Brian. (2018). Effects of fasted vs fed-state exercise on performance and post-exercise metabolism: A systematic review and meta-analysis. Scandinavian Journal of Medicine & Science in Sports. 28. 10.1111/sms.13054.

38. Costa, Ricardo & Snipe, Rhiannon & Kitic, Cecilia & Gibson, P. (2017). Systematic review: Exercise-induced gastrointestinal syndrome-implications for health and intestinal disease. Alimentary pharmacology & therapeutics. 46. 10.1111/apt.14157.

39. Benedict, C., Vogel, H., Jonas, W., Woting, A., Blaut, M., Schürmann, A., & Cedernaes, J. (2016). Gut microbiota and glucometabolic alterations in response to recurrent partial sleep deprivation in normal-weight young individuals. *Molecular metabolism,* 5(12), 1175–1186. doi:10.1016/j.molmet.2016.10.003

40. Centers for Disease Control. 2014. Short Sleep Duration Among US Adults. https://www.cdc.gov/sleep/data_statistics.html

41. Li, Y., Hao, Y., Fan, F., & Zhang, B. (2018). The Role of Microbiome in Insomnia, Circadian Disturbance and Depression. *Frontiers in psychiatry, 9,* 669. doi:10.3389/fpsyt.2018.00669

42. Williamson, A. M., & Feyer, A. M. (2000). Moderate sleep deprivation produces impairments in cognitive and motor performance equivalent to legally prescribed levels of alcohol intoxication. *Occupational and environmental medicine,* 57(10), 649–655. doi:10.1136/oem.57.10.649

43. Leproult, Rachel & Copinschi, Georges & Buxton, Orfeu & Van Cauter, Eve. (1997). Sleep Loss Results in an Elevation of Cortisol Levels the Next Evening. Sleep. 20. 865-70. 10.1093/sleep/20.10.865.

44. Karine Spiegel, Rachel Leproult, Mireille L'Hermite-Balériaux, Georges Copinschi, Plamen D. Penev, Eve Van Cauter, Leptin Levels Are Dependent on Sleep Duration: Relationships with Sympathovagal Balance, Carbohydrate Regulation, Cortisol, and Thyrotropin, *The Journal of Clinical Endocrinology & Metabolism,* Volume 89, Issue 11, 1 November 2004, Pages 5762–5771, https://doi.org/10.1210/jc.2004-1003

45. Taheri, S., Lin, L., Austin, D., Young, T., & Mignot, E. (2004). Short sleep duration is associated with reduced leptin, elevated ghrelin, and increased body mass index. *PLoS medicine, 1*(3), e62. doi:10.1371/journal.pmed.0010062

46. Mullington JM, Chan JL, Van Dongen HP, Szuba MP, Samaras J, Price NJ, Meier-Ewert HK, Dinges DF, Mantzoros CS. 2003. Sleep loss reduces diurnal rhythm amplitude of leptin in healthy men. Journal of Neuroendocrinology. Sep;15(9): 85; 1-4. https://www.ncbi.nlm.nih.gov/pubmed/12899679

47. Smith, R. P., Easson, C., Lyle, S. M., Kapoor, R., Donnelly, C. P., Davidson, E. J., ... Tartar, J. L. (2019). Gut microbiome diversity is associated with sleep physiology in humans. *PloS one, 14*(10), e0222394. doi:10.1371/journal.pone.0222394

48. Anderson, Jason & Carroll, Ian & Azcárate-Peril, Maria & Rochette, Amber & Heinberg, Leslie & Peat, Christine & Steffen, Kristine & Manderino, Lisa & Mitchell, James & Gunstad, John. (2017). A preliminary examination of gut microbiota, sleep, and cognitive flexibility in healthy older adults. Sleep Medicine. 38. 10.1016/j.sleep.2017.07.018.

49. Giau, V. V., Wu, S. Y., Jamerlan, A., An, S., Kim, S. Y., & Hulme, J. (2018). Gut Microbiota and Their Neuroinflammatory Implications in Alzheimer's Disease. *Nutrients, 10*(11), 1765. doi:10.3390/nu10111765

50. Belkaid, Y., & Hand, T. W. (2014). Role of the microbiota in immunity and inflammation. *Cell, 157*(1), 121–141. doi:10.1016/j.cell.2014.03.011

51. Krueger, J. M., Majde, J. A., & Rector, D. M. (2011). Cytokines in immune function and sleep regulation. *Handbook of clinical neurology, 98,* 229–240. doi:10.1016/B978-0-444-52006-7.00015-0

52. IY Chen, DC Jarrin, H Ivers, A Rochefort, CM Morin, 0291 ASSOCIATION BETWEEN STRESS-INDUCED AROUSAL AND NOCTURNAL SLEEP, *Sleep*, Volume 40, Issue suppl_1, 28 April 2017, Pages A107–A108, https://doi.org/10.1093/sleepj/zsx050.290

53. Sun, L., Zhang, X., Zhang, Y., Zheng, K., Xiang, Q., Chen, N., ... He, Q. (2019). Antibiotic-Induced Disruption of Gut Microbiota Alters Local Metabolomes and Immune Responses. *Frontiers in cellular and infection microbiology, 9*, 99. doi:10.3389/fcimb.2019.00099

54. Takada, M. & Nishida, Kensei & Gondo, Y. & Kikuchi-Hayakawa, H. & Ishikawa, H. & Kazunori, Suda & Kawai, Mitsuhisa & Hoshi, R. & Kuwano, Y. & Miyazaki, K. & Rokutan, K.. (2017). Beneficial effects of Lactobacillus casei strain Shirota on academic stress-induced sleep disturbance in healthy adults: A double-blind, randomised, placebo-controlled trial. Beneficial Microbes. 8. 153-162. 10.3920/BM2016.0150.

55. Thompson, R. S., Roller, R., Mika, A., Greenwood, B. N., Knight, R., Chichlowski, M., ... Fleshner, M. (2017). Dietary Prebiotics and Bioactive Milk Fractions Improve NREM Sleep, Enhance REM Sleep Rebound and Attenuate the Stress-Induced Decrease in Diurnal Temperature and Gut Microbial Alpha Diversity. *Frontiers in behavioral neuroscience, 10,* 240. doi:10.3389/fnbeh.2016.00240

56. Chi, Y. C., Sha, F., Yip, P. S., Chen, J. L., & Chen, Y. Y. (2016). Randomized comparison of group versus individual educational interventions for pregnant women to reduce their secondhand smoke exposure. *Medicine, 95*(40), e5072. doi:10.1097/MD.0000000000005072

57. Lax, S., Smith, D. P., Hampton-Marcell, J., Owens, S. M., Handley, K. M., Scott, N. M., ... Gilbert, J. A. (2014). Longitudinal analysis of microbial interaction between humans and the indoor environment. *Science (New York, N.Y.), 345*(6200), 1048–1052. doi:10.1126/science.1254529

58. Archie, Elizabeth & Theis, Kevin. (2011). Animal behavior meets microbial ecology. Animal Behaviour. 82. 425-436. 10.1016/j.anbehav.2011.05.029.

59. Xie, Lulu & Kang, Hongyi & Xu, Qiwu & Chen, Michael & Liao, Yonghong & Thiyagarajan, Meenakshisundaram & O'Donnell, John & Christensen, Daniel & Nicholson, Charles & Iliff, Jeffrey & Takano, Takahiro & Deane, Rashid & Nedergaard, Maiken. (2013). Sleep Drives Metabolite Clearance from the Adult Brain. Science (New York, N.Y.). 342. 373-7. 10.1126/science.1241224.

60. Everson, Carol & Bergmann, Bernard & Rechtschaffen, Allan. (1989). Sleep Deprivation in the Rat: III. Total Sleep Deprivation. Sleep. 12. 13-21. 10.1093/sleep/12.1.13.

61. Moeller, Andrew & Foerster, Steffen & Wilson, Michael & Pusey, Anne & Hahn, Beatrice & Ochman, Howard. (2016). Social behavior shapes the chimpanzee pan-microbiome. Science Advances. 2. e1500997-e1500997. 10.1126/sciadv.1500997.

62. House, James & Landis, Karl & Umberson, Debra. (1988). Social Relationships and Health. Science (New York, N.Y.). 241. 540-5. 10.1126/science.3399889.

63. Maher AC, *et al.* Psychological well-being in elderly adults with extraordinary episodic memory. PLoS One. 2017 Oct 23;12(10):e0186413.

64. Ellen Peters, J. Marianne Riksen-Walraven, Antonius H. N. Cillessen, Carolina de Weerth. Peer Rejection and HPA Activity in Middle Childhood: Friendship Makes a Difference. *Child Development*, 2011; DOI: 10.1111/j.1467-8624.2011.01647.x

65. Blue Cross BlueShield. 2019. The Health of Millennials. Blue Cross Blue Shield Health Index. https://www.bcbs.com/the-health-of-america/reports/the-health-of-millennials?utm_source=prnw&utm_medium=&utm_content=&utm_campaign=bcbs.com&utm_campaign=hoa_millhealth

66. Cigna. 2018. New Cigna Study Reveals Loneliness at Epidemic Levels in America. Cigna's Loneliness Survey. https://www.multivu.com/players/English/8294451-cigna-us-loneliness-survey/

67. Sharon, Gil & Segal, Daniel & Ringo, John & Hefetz, Abraham & Zilber-Rosenberg, Ilana & Rosenberg, Eugene. (2010). Commensal bacteria play a role in mating preference of Drosophila

melanogaster. Proceedings of the National Academy of Sciences of the United States of America. 107. 20051-6. 10.1073/pnas.1009906107.

68. Erdman, S.E. & Poutahidis, Theofilos. (2016). Microbes and Oxytocin: Benefits for Host Physiology and Behavior. 10.1016/bs.irn.2016.07.004.

69. Laura E. Grieneisen, Josh Livermore, Susan Alberts, Jenny Tung, Elizabeth A. Archie, Group Living and Male Dispersal Predict the Core Gut Microbiome in Wild Baboons, *Integrative and Comparative Biology,* Volume 57, Issue 4, October 2017, Pages 770–785, https://doi.org/10.1093/icb/icx046

70. Vuong, H. E., & Hsiao, E. Y. (2019). Gut Microbes Join the Social Network. *Neuron, 101*(2), 196–198. doi:10.1016/j.neuron.2018.12.035

71. Durk, R. P., Castillo, E., Márquez-Magaña, L., Grosicki, G. J., Bolter, N. D., Lee, C. M., & Bagley, J. R. (2019). Gut Microbiota Composition Is Related to Cardiorespiratory Fitness in Healthy Young Adults. *International journal of sport nutrition and exercise metabolism, 29*(3), 249–253. https://doi.org/10.1123/ijsnem.2018-0024

72. Dulai *et al.* 2018. Hyperbaric oxygen therapy is well tolerated and effective for ulcerative colitis patients hospitalized for moderate-severe flares: a phase 2A pilot multi-center, randomized, double-blind, sham-controlled trial. American Journal of Gastroenterology. Oct;113(10):1516-1523. doi: 10.1038/s41395-018-0005-z. Retrieved from: https://www.ncbi.nlm.nih.gov/pubmed/29453383.

73. Ng, Siew & Shi, Hai Yun & Hamidi, Nima & Underwood, Fox & Tang, Whitney & Benchimol, Eric & Panaccione, Remo & Ghosh, Subrata & Wu, Justin & Chan, Francis K.L. & Sung, Joseph & Kaplan, Gilaad. (2017). Worldwide incidence and prevalence of inflammatory bowel disease in the 21st century: A systematic review of population-based studies. The Lancet. 390. 10.1016/S0140-6736(17)32448-0.

74. Ouethrani M., Van de Wiele T., Verbeke E., Bruneau A., Carvalho M., Rabot S., *et al.* . (2013). Metabolic fate of ochratoxin A as a coffee contaminant in a dynamic simulator of the human colon. Food Chem. 141, 3291–3300. 10.1016/j.foodchem.2013.05.157

75. Taheri, Mahmoud & Mortazavi, SMJ & Moradi, Meysam & Mansouri, Shahla & Hatam, Gholam Reza & Nouri, Fateme. (2017). Evaluation of the Effect of Radiofrequency Radiation Emitted From Wi-Fi Router and Mobile Phone Simulator on the Antibacterial Susceptibility of Pathogenic Bacteria Listeria monocytogenes and Escherichia coli. Dose-Response. 15. 155932581668852. 10.1177/1559325816688527.

76. Nascimento, Luiz & Botura Junior, Galdenoro & Mota, Rogério. (2003). Glucose consume and growth of E. coli Under electromagnetic field. Revista do Instituto de Medicina Tropical de São Paulo. 45. 65-7. 10.1590/S0036-46652003000200002.

77. Garg, Akshay & Vasistha, Sharsti. (2016). Effect of Electromagnetic radiation on Lactobacillus species. Journal of Chemical and Pharmaceutical Research. Journal of Chemical and Pharmaceutical Research. 8.

78. Nathan, Neil. 2018. Toxic: Heal Your Body from Mold Toxicity, Lyme Disease, Multiple Chemical Sensitivities, and Chronic Environmental Illness. Victory Belt Publishing.

79. Tenk, E. Fodor, C. Szathmáry. The effect of pure Fusarium toxins (T-2, F-2, DAS) on the microflora of the gut and on plasma glucocorticoid levels in rats and swine. Zentralbl Bakteriol Mikrobiol Hyg A, 252 (1982), pp. 384-393.

80. Li, Y. T., Xu, H., Ye, J. Z., Wu, W. R., Shi, D., Fang, D. Q., Liu, Y., & Li, L. J. (2019). Efficacy of *Lactobacillus rhamnosus* GG in treatment of acute pediatric diarrhea: A systematic review with meta-analysis. *World journal of gastroenterology, 25*(33), 4999–5016. https://doi.org/10.3748/wjg.v25.i33.4999

81. Buffington, S. A., Di Prisco, G. V., Auchtung, T. A., Ajami, N. J., Petrosino, J. F., & Costa-Mattioli, M. (2016). Microbial Reconstitution Reverses Maternal Diet-Induced Social and Synaptic Deficits in Offspring. *Cell, 165*(7), 1762–1775. https://doi.org/10.1016/j.cell.2016.06.001

82. Venu, Isvarya & Durisko, Zachary & Xu, Jianping & Dukas, Reuven. (2014). Social attraction mediated by fruit flies' microbiome. The Journal of experimental biology. 217. 1346-52. 10.1242/jeb.099648.

83. Erdman, S.E. & Poutahidis, Theofilos. (2016). Microbes and Oxytocin: Benefits for Host Physiology and Behavior. 10.1016/bs.irn.2016.07.004.

84. Claesson, M. J., Jeffery, I. B., Conde, S., Power, S. E., O'Connor, E. M., Cusack, S., ... O'Toole, P. W. (2012). Gut microbiota compo- sition correlates with diet and health in the elderly. *Nature*, **488**, 178–184. doi:10.1038/nature11319

85. Martins IJ. Overnutrition Determines LPS Regulation of Mycotoxin Induced Neurotoxicity in Neurodegenerative Diseases. *Int J Mol Sci.* 2015;16(12):29554-29573. Published 2015 Dec 10. doi:10.3390/ijms161226190

86. Laurent, H. K., Stroud, L. R., Brush, B., D'Angelo, C., & Granger, D. A. (2015). Secretory IgA reactivity to social threat in youth: Relations with HPA, ANS, and behavior. Psychoneuroendocrinology, 59, 81–90. https://doi.org/10.1016/j.psyneuen.2015.04.021

87. Kuo B, Bhasin M, Jacquart J, *et al.* Genomic and clinical effects associated with a relaxation response mind-body intervention in patients with irritable bowel syndrome and inflammatory bowel disease [published correction appears in PLoS One. 2017 Feb 21;12 (2):e0172872]. *PLoS One.* 2015;10(4):e0123861. Published 2015 Apr 30. doi:10.1371/journal.pone.0123861

88. González-Moret, R., Cebolla, A., Cortés, X., Baños, R. M., Navarrete, J., de la Rubia, J. E., Lisón, J. F., & Soria, J. M. (2020). The effect of a mindfulness-based therapy on different biomarkers among patients with inflammatory bowel disease: a randomised controlled trial. *Scientific Reports, 10*(1), 6071. https://doi-org.uws.idm.oclc.org/10.1038/s41598-020-63168-4

89. Emmons RA, McCullough ME. Counting blessings versus burdens: an experimental investigation of gratitude and subjective well-being in daily life. J Pers Soc Psychol. 2003;84(2):377-389. doi:10.1037//0022-3514.84.2.377

90. Morgan, N., Irwin, M. R., Chung, M., & Wang, C. (2014). The effects of mind-body therapies on the immune system: meta-analysis. PloS one, 9(7), e100903. https://doi.org/10.1371/journal.pone.0100903

91. Davidson RJ, Kabat-Zinn J, Schumacher J, Rosenkranz M, Muller D, *et al.* (2003) Alterations in brain and immune function produced by mindfulness meditation. Psychosom Med 65: 564–570.

92. Korb, Alex. 2015. The Upward Spiral: Using Neuroscience to Reverse the Course of Depression, One Small Change at a Time. New Harbinger Publications.

93. Huo R, Zeng B, Zeng L, *et al.* Microbiota Modulate Anxiety-Like Behavior and Endocrine Abnormalities in Hypothalamic-Pituitary-Adrenal Axis. Front Cell Infect Microbiol. 2017;7:489. Published 2017 Nov 30. doi:10.3389/fcimb.2017.00489

94. Redwine LS, Henry BL, Pung MA, *et al.* Pilot Randomized Study of a Gratitude Journaling Intervention on Heart Rate Variability and Inflammatory Biomarkers in Patients With Stage B Heart Failure. Psychosom Med. 2016;78(6):667-676. doi:10.1097/PSY.0000000000000316

95. Brown, S. R., Cann, P. A., & Read, N. W. (1990). Effect of coffee on distal colon function. *Gut, 31*(4), 450–453. https://doi.org/10.1136/gut.31.4.450

96. Mann T, Tomiyama AJ, Westling E, Lew AM, Samuels B, Chatman J. Medicare's search for effective obesity treatments: diets are not the answer. *Am Psychol.* 2007;62(3):220-233. doi:10.1037/0003-066X.62.3.220

97. CDC. 2017. Only 1 in 10 adults gets enough fruits and vegetables. https://www.cdc.gov/media/releases/2017/p1116-fruit-vegetable-consumption.html

98. Duncan SH, Belenguer A, Holtrop G, Johnstone AM, Flint HJ, Lobley GE. Reduced dietary intake of carbohydrates by obese subjects results in decreased concentrations of butyrate and

butyrate-producing bacteria in feces. *Appl Environ Microbiol*. 2007;73(4):1073-1078. doi:10.1128/AEM.02340-06

99. Proctor, L.M., Creasy, H.H., Fettweis, J.M. *et al.* The Integrative Human Microbiome Project. *Nature* **569**, 641–648 (2019). https://doi.org/10.1038/s41586-019-1238-8

100. Mohr, A.E., Jäger, R., Carpenter, K.C. *et al.* The athletic gut microbiota. *J Int Soc Sports Nutr* **17**, 24 (2020). https://doi.org/10.1186/s12970-020-00353-w

101. Aguilera M., Vergara P., Martinez V. Stress and antibiotics alter luminal and wall-adhered microbiota and enhance the local expression of visceral sensory-related systems in mice. Neurogastroenterology Motility. 2013;25:e515–e529.

102. Tannock G.W., Savage D.C. Influences of dietary and environmental stress on microbial populations in the murine gastrointestinal tract. Infect Immun. 1974;9:591–598.

103. Zijlmans M.A., Korpela K., Riksen-Walraven J.M., de Vos W.M., de Weerth C. Maternal prenatal stress is associated with the infant intestinal microbiota. Psychoneuroendocrinology. 2015;53:233–245.

104. Niranga Manjuri Devanarayana, Shaman Rajindrajith, Association between Constipation and Stressful Life Events in a Cohort of Sri Lankan Children and Adolescents, *Journal of Tropical Pediatrics*, Volume 56, Issue 3, June 2010, Pages 144–148, https://doi.org/10.1093/tropej/fmp077

105. Cignarella, F., Cantoni, C., Ghezzi, L., Salter, A., Dorsett, Y., Chen, L., Phillips, D., Weinstock, G. M., Fontana, L., Cross, A. H., Zhou, Y., & Piccio, L. (2018). Intermittent Fasting Confers Protection in CNS Autoimmunity by Altering the Gut Microbiota. *Cell metabolism, 27*(6), 1222–1235.e6. https://doi.org/10.1016/j.cmet.2018.05.006

106. Li, L., Su, Y., Li, F. *et al.* The effects of daily fasting hours on shaping gut microbiota in mice. *BMC Microbiol* **20**, 65 (2020). https://doi.org/10.1186/s12866-020-01754-2

107. He, Yan & Yin, Jia & Lei, Jun & Liu, Feitong & Zheng, Huimin & Wang, Shan & Wu, Shan & Sheng, Huafang & Mcgovern, Emily & Zhou, Hongwei. (2019). Fasting Challenges Human Gut Microbiome Resilience and Reduces Fusobacterium. Medicine in Microecology. 1-2. 100003. 10.1016/j.medmic.2019.100003.

108. Gabel, K., Marcell, J., Cares, K., Kalam, F., Cienfuegos, S., Ezpeleta, M., & Varady, K. A. (2020). Effect of time restricted feeding on the gut microbiome in adults with obesity: A pilot study. *Nutrition and Health*. https://doi.org/10.1177/0260106020910907

109. Cattaneo, C., Gargari, G., Koirala, R. *et al.* New insights into the relationship between taste perception and oral microbiota composition. *Sci Rep* **9**, 3549 (2019). https://doi.org/10.1038/s41598-019-40374-3

110. Parkar, S., Kalsbeek, A., & Cheeseman, J. (2019). Potential Role for the Gut Microbiota in Modulating Host Circadian Rhythms and Metabolic Health. *Microorganisms, 7*(2), 41. MDPI AG. Retrieved from http://dx.doi.org/10.3390/microorganisms7020041

111. Benedict, C., Vogel, H., Jonas, W., Woting, A., Blaut, M., Schürmann, A., & Cedernaes, J. (2016). Gut microbiota and glucometabolic alterations in response to recurrent partial sleep deprivation in normal-weight young individuals. *Molecular metabolism,* 5(12), 1175–1186. https://doi.org/10.1016/j.molmet.2016.10.003

112. Hirano, Arisa & Hsu, Pei-Ken & Zhang, Luoying & Xing, Lijuan & McMahon, Thomas & Yamazaki, Maya & Ptácek, Louis & Fu, Ying-Hui. (2018). DEC2 modulates orexin expression and regulates sleep. Proceedings of the National Academy of Sciences. 115. 201801693. 10.1073/pnas.1801693115.

113. Demarinis S. Loneliness at epidemic levels in America. Explore (NY). 2020 Sep-Oct;16(5):278-279. doi: 10.1016/j.explore.2020.06.008. Epub 2020 Jun 28. PMID: 32674944; PMCID: PMC7321652.

114. Wedekind C, Seebeck T, Bettens F, Paepke AJ. MHC-dependent mate preferences in humans. Proc Biol Sci. 1995 Jun 22;260(1359):245-9. doi: 10.1098/rspb.1995.0087. PMID: 7630893.

115. Tarazona, A., Gómez, J. V., Mateo, F., Jiménez, M., & Mateo, E. M. (2021). Potential Health Risk Associated with Mycotoxins in Oat Grains Consumed in Spain. *Toxins, 13*(6). https://doi-org.uws.idm.oclc.org/10.3390/toxins13060421

116. Del Castilo, I., Neumann, A. S., Lemos, F. S., De Bastiani, M. A., Oliveira, F. L., Zimmer, E. R., Rêgo, A. M., Hardoim, C. C. P., Antunes, L. C. M., Lara, F. A., Figueiredo, C. P., & Clarke, J. R (2022). Lifelong Exposure to a Low-Dose of the Glyphosate-Based Herbicide RoundUp ® Causes Intestinal Damage, Gut Dysbiosis, and Behavioral Changes in Mice. *International Journal of Molecular Sciences, 23*(10), 5583. https://doi-org.uws.idm.oclc.org/10.3390/ijms23105583

117. Ehrenstein, Ondine & Ling, Chenxiao & Cui, Xin & Cockburn, Myles & Park, Andrew & Yu, Fei & Wu, Jun & Ritz, Beate. (2019). Prenatal and infant exposure to ambient pesticides and autism spectrum disorder in children: Population based case-control study. BMJ. 364. l962. 10.1136/bmj.l962.

118. Hyslop, G. (2022, April 20). Consumer knowledge about glyphosate-tainted foods still 'dangerously' lacking. *Global Food.*

119. Kim, E. S., Chen, Y., Nakamura, J. S., Ryff, C. D., & VanderWeele, T. J. (2022). Sense of Purpose in Life and Subsequent Physical, Behavioral, and Psychosocial Health: An Outcome-Wide Approach. *American Journal of Health Promotion, 36*(1), 137–147.

# PART FOUR: WHAT NEXT?

# CHAPTER 19:
# TRUST YOUR GUT.

Final Destination: Trust your gut.

Now that you know how to tune in to your current gut health and how to take care of your gut with your inner Eight Superpowers and customized nutrition and supplements, let's get to the "secret sauce" for a Total Gut Reset—trust your gut.

Trusting your gut is the secret sauce for less stress overall.

## TRUST YOUR GUT

You were born with the innate ability to "go with your gut." Intuition.

Intuition means the ability to understand something immediately, without the need for conscious reasoning. Whether you call it a gut feeling, an inner voice, or a sixth sense, intuition can play a real part in our daily lifestyle choices and all-around health.

Tons of research actually suggests that our ability to repeatedly exert self-control (over our gut intuition) is actually quite limited. Like a muscle that tires and can no longer perform at its peak strength after a workout, our self-control is diminished by previous efforts at control, even if those efforts take place in a totally different realm.

Not going with your gut will burn you out, stress you out and not make you well. Listening to your gut on the other hand—from deciding what foods work best for you to saying "no" instead of saying yes all the time—makes you more confident and can actually propel you to feeling better overall.

In an experiment of college students, participants were shown images of a cloud of many moving dots, which looked like the noisy "snow" you might see on an old TV. Participants had to report which general direction the cloud of dots was moving in: left or right.

While subjects made these decisions, researchers presented one of their eyes with emotional photographs (positive images like puppies and negative images like snakes) through a technique called "continuous flash suppression," making the emotional photographs invisible or unconscious. In short: While the subjects made their sensory decisions, they never knew they were being presented with the emotional photographs.

In all four different experiments, researchers found that people were able to make faster and more accurate decisions when they unconsciously viewed the emotional images. Essentially, people's brains were able to process and utilize information from the images to intuitively go with their gut feelings and improve their decisions. Moreover, participants got faster as the study went on, suggesting practice—and giving yourself permission to go with your gut—makes it easier and *better.*

Other research shows that we become *more* stressed when we *don't* go with our gut, and over time, we eventually just can't do it; we cave, and we fall apart inside. One study of college students showed the obvious: engaging in self-weighing and calorie counting (going *against* your gut intuition and pushing yourself to chisel your body harder) resulted in elevated disordered eating and full-blown eating disorders compared to those who were taught the skills of intuitive eating. Another study investigating what happens when we actually *do* listen to our gut found that when people are given permission to go with their gut (i.e., do the right thing), their physical health improves. In the study, researchers simply educated subjects in the art of being honest and gave them permission to listen to their gut intuition—tell *lies* less often in the day. As a result, all subjects reported significant increases in their confidence and overall sense of well-being.

## TRUSTING MY GUT (IN REAL LIFE)

I'll never forget the day that I decided to withdraw my application from medical school because I was already doing what I loved.

And I'll never forget the day that I threw away all the supplements that weren't helping me.

Or the day that I decided to stop counting calories or fearing food and ordering what sounded good on the menu.

And the day that I let my body sleep, waking up at 7 a.m. instead of my usual 5:30 a.m. because it needed it.

I'll never forget the time that I said "no" to overcommitting myself for the 20th time in a row.

Or the time that I ate beef for the first time in ten years, knowing my body was craving it.

I'll never forget the time that I said "yes" and hired the new employee who was the perfect candidate for the job.

And I'll never forget the butterflies I had when I was around that guy—but not another (my microbes know what they like).

Trusting your gut is one of the greatest things you can do to reclaim balance from the inside out. Less stress. Especially once your "Gut Love Superpowers" are in place.

It's one thing to be eating Doritos, hydrating with 3-4 cups of coffee, couch surfing every single day, and "trusting your gut", versus having a healthier baseline upon which to take your cues—especially since the gut is connected to your brain!

## REWIRE THE GUT-BRAIN CONNECTION

Oh yes. The Gut-Brain Connection. Really, **trusting your gut** is all about rewiring the Gut-Brain Connection and how you think and feel by *actually* trusting your gut instead of worrying, stressing, or overthinking.

Vanessa is a perfect example.

Vanessa, 55, was a Hollywood hairdresser who, like many, could not lose those last 20 pounds. She tried everything, and nothing helped *until* she stopped diet hopping *and* quit her high-stress director position behind the scenes of the latest *Batman* movie. She trusted her gut. The pounds magically fell off, and her bloating and sugar cravings went away!

Then there was Ali, a 34-year-old mom of two. Ali had a former health history of anorexia, bulimia, three open heart surgeries, colitis, hypothyroidism, and recurring SIBO. Her diet consisted of about ten foods: gluten-free, dairy-free, soy-free, FODMAP-free, starch-free, histamine free, and most of her free time was dedicated to health-related podcasts and Dr. Google articles. All she wanted to do was "be normal." Enter: Her son's 4th birthday. Ali made him a cake with one intention: She would eat it. Even if she had a flare-up, she didn't care. Ali just wanted to experience his birthday *with* him. She ate a slice and, to her surprise, nothing happened. She was shocked!

Bill, 48, had IBS, anxiety, and bloating his entire life. After receiving his latest food intolerance results before a trip of a lifetime to Italy with his wife to celebrate their 20th anniversary, he freaked out, having no idea what she would eat. I gave him just two assignments: no email checking and, when in Rome, try some real pasta, which he did, for the first time in ten years. Surprisingly, no symptoms. The entire trip.

Or you may be like 23-year-old Lauryn. Me, at 79 pounds, and for the first time, scared for my life. Driving to the gym at 4 a.m., I prayed, "God help me make a change today." I didn't make it to my workout. Instead, nine "YMCA Angels" said they wanted to help. Within hours, I was at that hospital, doctors saying I may not make it. But amidst the chaos, something inside me knew it was going to be ok...I realized I was getting a new opportunity to start trusting my gut again so I could help others one day do the same.

Here's your permission: Listen (and go) with your gut.

## THE GUT CHECK METHOD

Above all, when in doubt, press pause and hone in on the good ol' *Gut Check Method* by asking yourself these simple questions.

*How do I feel?*
*Why do I feel this way?*
*What do I need?*

## GUT CHECK-IN

Find a quiet place to sit still for one minute. Close your eyes. Practice that deep, nose-based belly breathing. Check-in—with your body.

How do you feel, right now, in this moment?

Stomach settled and calm? Uncomfortable or irritated?
Slightly lightheaded—it's been a minute since you ate something?
Dry mouth?
Tight muscles?
Energized? Depleted from 6 hours of sleep last night?
Calm and peace?
Refreshed and nourished?
Brain foggy?

If something is off, the follow-up question is then to ask: *Why do I feel this way?* Then the best question of all: *What do I need?*

You were born with the innate ability to "go with your gut."

### RESOURCES


1. Donkin, Chris. (2016). Measuring intuition: Nonconscious emotional information boosts decision accuracy and confidence. Psychological Science.
2. Romano, K. A., Swanbrow Becker, M. A., Colgary, C. D., & Magnuson, A. (2018). Helpful or harmful? The comparative value of self-weighing and calorie counting versus intuitive eating on the eating disorder symptomology of college students. Eating and Weight Disorders – Studies on Anorexia, Bulimia and Obesity. doi:10.1007/s40519-018-0562-6
3. Kelly, A. E., & Wang, L. (2012). Lying Less Linked to Better Health, New Research Finds. Retrieved January 29, 2020, from https://www.apa.org/news/press/releases/2012/08/lying-less


### REFERENCES


1. Center for Disease Control. 2019. Chronic Diseases in America. https://www.cdc.gov/chronicdisease/resources/infographic/chronic-diseases.htm
2. Joana Araújo, Jianwen Cai, June Stevens. Prevalence of Optimal Metabolic Health in American Adults: National Health and Nutrition Examination Survey 2009–2016. *Metabolic Syndrome and Related Disorders*, 2018; DOI: 10.1089/met.2018.0105

3. Davis C. D. (2016). The Gut Microbiome and Its Role in Obesity. *Nutrition today, 51*(4), 167–174. doi:10.1097/NT.0000000000000167

4. Cattaneo, C., Gargari, G., Koirala, R. *et al.* New insights into the relationship between taste perception and oral microbiota composition. *Sci Rep* **9**, 3549 (2019). https://doi.org/10.1038/s41598-019-40374-3

5. Alcock, J., Maley, C. C., & Aktipis, C. A. (2014). Is eating behavior manipulated by the gastrointestinal microbiota? Evolutionary pressures and potential mechanisms. *BioEssays : news and reviews in molecular, cellular and developmental biology, 36*(10), 940–949. https://doi.org/10.1002/bies.201400071

6. A.K. Abbas, A.H.H. Lichtman, S. Pillai, Cellular and Molecular Immunology E-Book, Elsevier Health Sciences, 2017.

7. Stahnisch, F. W., & Verhoef, M. (2012). The flexner report of 1910 and its impact on complementary and alternative medicine and psychiatry in North America in the 20th century. *Evidence-based complementary and alternative medicine : eCAM, 2012,* 647896. https://doi.org/10.1155/2012/647896

8. A.K. Abbas, A.H.H. Lichtman, S. Pillai, Cellular and Molecular Immunology E-Book, Elsevier Health Sciences, 2017.

9. Froehlich, Eleonore & Wahl, Richard. (2019). Microbiota and Thyroid Interaction in Health and Disease. Trends in Endocrinology & Metabolism. 30. 10.1016/j.tem.2019.05.008.

10. Baker, James & Al-Nakkash, Layla & Herbst-Kralovetz, Melissa. (2017). Estrogen–Gut Microbiome Axis: Physiological and Clinical Implications. Maturitas. 103. 10.1016/j.maturitas.2017.06.025.

11. Tremellen, K., McPhee, N., Pearce, K., Benson, S., Schedlowski, M., & Engler, H. (2018). Endotoxin-initiated inflammation reduces testosterone production in men of reproductive age. *American journal of physiology. Endocrinology and metabolism, 314*(3), E206–E213. doi:10.1152/ajpendo.00279.2017

12. Martin, C. R., Osadchiy, V., Kalani, A., & Mayer, E. A. (2018). The Brain-Gut-Microbiome Axis. *Cellular and molecular gastroenterology and hepatology, 6*(2), 133–148. doi:10.1016/j.jcmgh.2018.04.003

13. Thomas C. Fung, Helen E. Vuong, Cristopher D. G. Luna, Geoffrey N. Pronovost, Antoniya A. Aleksandrova, Noah G. Riley, Anastasia Vavilina, Julianne McGinn, Tomiko Rendon, Lucy R. Forrest, Elaine Y. Hsiao. Intestinal serotonin and fluoxetine exposure modulate bacterial colonization in the gut. *Nature Microbiology*, 2019; DOI: 10.1038/s41564-019-0540-4

14. Lyte M. (2013). Microbial endocrinology in the microbiome-gut-brain axis: how bacterial production and utilization of neurochemicals influence behavior. *PLoS pathogens, 9*(11), e1003726. doi:10.1371/journal.ppat.1003726

15. Serge Rezzi, Ziad Ramadan, François-Pierre J. Martin, Laurent B. Fay, Peter van Bladeren, John C. Lindon, Jeremy K. Nicholson, and, and Sunil Kochhar. (2007) Human Metabolic Phenotypes Link Directly to Specific Dietary Preferences in Healthy Individuals. Journal of Proteome Research. 6 (11), 4469-4477. DOI: 10.1021/pr070431h

16. Kalliomäki, Marko & Collado, Maria Carmen & Salminen, Seppo & Isolauri, Erika. (2008). Early differences in fecal microbiota composition in children may predict overweight. The American journal of clinical nutrition. 87. 534-8. 10.1093/ajcn/87.3.534.

17. Depommier C, Everard A, Druart C, *et al.* Supplementation with Akkermansia muciniphila in overweight and obese human volunteers: a proof-of-concept exploratory study. Nat Med. 2019. doi: 10.1038/s41591-019-0495-2.

18. Centers for Disease Control. 2019. Chronic Diseases in America. https://www.cdc.gov/chronicdisease/resources/infographic/chronic-diseases.htm

19. Kotzampassi, Katerina. (2013). Bacteria and Obesity: The Proportion Makes the Difference. Surgery: Current Research. 03. 10.4172/2161-1076.1000152.

20. Fox News. 2015. Survey shows 74 percent of Americans living with GI discomfort. Retrieved from: https://www.foxnews.com/health/survey-shows-74-percent-of-americans-living-with-gi-discomfort

21. Segata N. Gut Microbiome: Westernization and the Disappearance of Intestinal Diversity. *Curr Biol.* 2015;25(14):R611-R613. doi:10.1016/j.cub.2015.05.040

22. Fothergill, E., Guo, J., Howard, L., Kerns, J. C., Knuth, N. D., Brychta, R., ... Hall, K. D. (2016). Persistent metabolic adaptation 6 years after "The Biggest Loser" competition. *Obesity (Silver Spring, Md.), 24*(8), 1612–1619. doi:10.1002/oby.21538

23. Rogers, G. B., Keating, D. J., Young, R. L., Wong, M. L., Licinio, J., & Wesselingh, S. (2016). From gut dysbiosis to altered brain function and mental illness: mechanisms and pathways. *Molecular psychiatry, 21*(6), 738–748. doi:10.1038/mp.2016.50

24. Jim E. Banta, Gina Segovia-Siapco, Christine Betty Crocker, Danielle Montoya, Noara Alhusseini. Mental health status and dietary intake among California adults: a population-based survey. *International Journal of Food Sciences and Nutrition,* 2019; 1 DOI: 10.1080/09637486.2019.1570085

25. Wu, G. D., Chen, J., Hoffmann, C., Bittinger, K., Chen, Y. Y., Keilbaugh, S. A., ... Lewis, J. D. (2011). Linking long-term dietary patterns with gut microbial enterotypes. *Science (New York, N.Y.), 334*(6052), 105–108. doi:10.1126/science.1208344

26. Cattaneo, Camilla & Gargari, Giorgio & Koirala, Ranjan & Laureati, M. & Riso, Patrizia & Guglielmetti, Simone & Pagliarini, Ella. (2019). New insights into the relationship between taste perception and oral microbiota composition. Scientific Reports. 9. 3549. 10.1038/s41598-019-40374-3.

27. Sergi, Giuseppe & Bano, Giulia & Pizzato, Simona & Veronese, Nicola & Manzato, Enzo. (2016). Taste Loss in the Elderly: Possible Implications for Dietary Habits. Critical reviews in food science and nutrition. 57. 10.1080/10408398.2016.1160208.

28. Nagpal, R., Mainali, R., Ahmadi, S., Wang, S., Singh, R., Kavanagh, K., ... Yadav, H. (2018). Gut microbiome and aging: Physiological and mechanistic insights. *Nutrition and healthy aging, 4*(4), 267–285. doi:10.3233/NHA-170030

29. Nagpal, R., Mainali, R., Ahmadi, S., Wang, S., Singh, R., Kavanagh, K., ... Yadav, H. (2018). Gut microbiome and aging: Physiological and mechanistic insights. *Nutrition and healthy aging, 4*(4), 267–285. doi:10.3233/NHA-170030

30. Garcia-Burgos, D., Maglieri, S., Vögele, C., & Munsch, S. (2018). How Does Food Taste in Anorexia and Bulimia Nervosa? A Protocol for a Quasi-Experimental, Cross-Sectional Design to Investigate Taste Aversion or Increased Hedonic Valence of Food in Eating Disorders. *Frontiers in psychology, 9,* 264. doi:10.3389/fpsyg.2018.00264

31. Seitz, J., Belheouane, M., Schulz, N., Dempfle, A., Baines, J. F., & Herpertz-Dahlmann, B. (2019). The Impact of Starvation on the Microbiome and Gut-Brain Interaction in Anorexia Nervosa. *Frontiers in endocrinology, 10,* 41. doi:10.3389/fendo.2019.00041

32. Glenny, E. M., Bulik-Sullivan, E. C., Tang, Q., Bulik, C. M., & Carroll, I. M. (2017). Eating Disorders and the Intestinal Microbiota: Mechanisms of Energy Homeostasis and Behavioral Influence. *Current psychiatry reports, 19*(8), 51. doi:10.1007/s11920-017-0797-3

RESOURCES:

# TUNE IN TO YOUR GUT BASELINE ASSESSMENTS

## ASSESSMENT #1: IDENTIFY YOUR GUT TYPE

**List your five major health concerns in order of importance, according to their primary symptoms** *(this is good to come back to after you implement a protocol).*

1.

2.

3.

4.

5.

**Check the appropriate number on all questions below, using zero as least/never and three as most/always.**

| Category 1 (Large Intestine Dysfunction: Colon Dysbiosis, Bacteria, or Yeast Overgrowth) | 0 | 1 | 2 | 3 |
|---|---|---|---|---|
| Feeling that bowels do not empty completely | ○ | ○ | ○ | ○ |
| Lower abdominal pain relieved by passing stool or gas | ○ | ○ | ○ | ○ |
| Alternating constipation and diarrhea | ○ | ○ | ○ | ○ |
| Diarrhea | ○ | ○ | ○ | ○ |
| Constipation | ○ | ○ | ○ | ○ |
| Hard, dry, or small stool | ○ | ○ | ○ | ○ |
| Coated tongue or fuzzy debris on tongue | ○ | ○ | ○ | ○ |
| Pass large amount of foul-smelling gas | ○ | ○ | ○ | ○ |
| More than three bowel movements daily | ○ | ○ | ○ | ○ |
| Use laxatives frequently | ○ | ○ | ○ | ○ |

| Category 2 (Small Intestinal Dysfunction: Leaky Gut, Fungal Overgrowth, & Dysbiosis) | 0 | 1 | 2 | 3 |
|---|---|---|---|---|
| Increasing frequency of food reactions | | | | |
| Unpredictable food reactions | | | | |
| Aches, pains, swelling, and/or inflammation in the body | | | | |
| Unpredictable abdominal swelling | | | | |
| Frequent bloating/distention after eating | | | | |
| Abdominal intolerance to sugars and starches | | | | |
| Sometimes feel better when you don't eat | | | | |
| Mood imbalances (anxiety, depression, etc.) | | | | |
| Skin breakouts (eczema, zits, dry flaky skin) | | | | |
| Headaches, brain fog, or memory loss | | | | |
| Low immunity (allergies, easily sick) | | | | |

| Category 3 (Upper GI Imbalance: Low Stomach Acid, Possible SIBO) | 0 | 1 | 2 | 3 |
|---|---|---|---|---|
| Excessive belching, burping, or bloating | ○ | ○ | ○ | ○ |
| Gas immediately following a meal | ○ | ○ | ○ | ○ |
| Offensive breath | ○ | ○ | ○ | ○ |
| Difficult bowel movement | ○ | ○ | ○ | ○ |
| Sense of fullness during and after meals | ○ | ○ | ○ | ○ |
| Difficulty digesting fruits and vegetables; undigested food found in stools | ○ | ○ | ○ | ○ |

| Category 4 (Stomach, GERD) | 0 | 1 | 2 | 3 |
|---|---|---|---|---|
| Stomach pain, burning, or aching one to four hours after eating | ○ | ○ | ○ | ○ |
| Use antacids | ○ | ○ | ○ | ○ |
| Feel hungry an hour or two after eating | ○ | ○ | ○ | ○ |
| Heartburn when lying down or bending forward | ○ | ○ | ○ | ○ |
| Temporary relief by using antacids, food, milk, or carbonated beverages | ○ | ○ | ○ | ○ |
| Digestive problems subside with rest and relaxation | ○ | ○ | ○ | ○ |
| Heartburn due to spicy foods, chocolate, citrus, peppers, alcohol, and caffeine | ○ | ○ | ○ | ○ |

| Category 5 (Small Intestine, SIBO) | 0 | 1 | 2 | 3 |
|---|---|---|---|---|
| Abdominal distention after consumption of fiber, starch, and/or sugar | | | | |
| Frequent gas | | | | |
| Probiotics or natural supplements cause bloating | | | | |
| Lowered GI motility, constipation | | | | |
| Raised GI motility, diarrhea | | | | |
| Alternating constipation and diarrhea | | | | |
| Suspect nutritional malabsorption | | | | |
| Unwanted weight loss or weight gain | | | | |
| Frequent use of antacid medication | | | | |

| | | | | |
|---|---|---|---|---|
| Skin breakouts (eczema, zits, dry flaky skin) | | | | |
| Headaches, brain fog, or memory loss | | | | |
| History of diagnosis of celiac disease, IBS, diverticulosis/diverticulitis, or leaky gut | | | | |
| History of birth control use (0=never, 1=over 5 years ago, 2=within past 5 years, 3=currently taking) | ○ | ○ | ○ | ○ |
| Fat malabsorption (greasy, pale, or bulky stools) | ○ | ○ | ○ | ○ |
| Food intolerances (gluten, casein, lactose, fructose) | ○ | ○ | ○ | ○ |
| Sensitive/reactive to high histamine foods (bone broth, avocado, spinach, fermented foods, chocolate, leftover meat, seafood, citrus, berries) | ○ | ○ | ○ | ○ |
| Autoimmune disease (0=no, 3=yes) | ○ | ○ | ○ | ○ |

| **Category 6 (Pancreas)** | **0** | **1** | **2** | **3** |
|---|---|---|---|---|
| Roughage and fiber cause constipation | ○ | ○ | ○ | ○ |
| Indigestion and fullness last two to four hours after eating | ○ | ○ | ○ | ○ |
| Pain, tenderness, soreness on left side under rib cage | ○ | ○ | ○ | ○ |
| Excessive passage of gas | ○ | ○ | ○ | ○ |
| Nausea and/or vomiting | ○ | ○ | ○ | ○ |
| Stool contains undigested food, is foul smelling, mucous-like, greasy, or poorly formed | ○ | ○ | ○ | ○ |
| Frequent urination | ○ | ○ | ○ | ○ |
| Increased thirst and appetite | ○ | ○ | ○ | ○ |

| **Category 7 (Gallbladder)** | **0** | **1** | **2** | **3** |
|---|---|---|---|---|
| Greasy or high-fat foods cause distress | ○ | ○ | ○ | ○ |
| Lower bowel gas and/or bloating several hours after eating | ○ | ○ | ○ | ○ |
| Bitter metallic taste in mouth, especially in the morning | ○ | ○ | ○ | ○ |
| Burpy, fishy taste after consuming fish oils | ○ | ○ | ○ | ○ |

| | | | | |
|---|---|---|---|---|
| Difficulty losing weight | ○ | ○ | ○ | ○ |
| Unexplained itchy skin | ○ | ○ | ○ | ○ |
| Yellowish cast to eyes | ○ | ○ | ○ | ○ |
| Stool color alternates from clay colored to normal brown | ○ | ○ | ○ | ○ |
| Reddened skin, especially palms | ○ | ○ | ○ | ○ |
| Dry or flaky skin and/or hair | ○ | ○ | ○ | ○ |
| History of gallbladder attacks or stones | ○ | ○ | ○ | ○ |
| Have you had your gallbladder removed? | ○ Yes | | ○ No | |

| **Category 8 (Liver)** | **0** | **1** | **2** | **3** |
|---|---|---|---|---|
| Acne and unhealthy skin | ○ | ○ | ○ | ○ |
| Excessive hair loss | ○ | ○ | ○ | ○ |
| Overall sense of bloating | ○ | ○ | ○ | ○ |
| Bodily swelling for no reason | ○ | ○ | ○ | ○ |
| Hormone imbalances | ○ | ○ | ○ | ○ |
| Weight gain | ○ | ○ | ○ | ○ |
| Poor bowel function | ○ | ○ | ○ | ○ |
| Excessively foul-smelling sweat | ○ | ○ | ○ | ○ |

| **Category 9 (Low Blood Sugar/Hypoglycemia)** | **0** | **1** | **2** | **3** |
|---|---|---|---|---|
| Crave sweets during the day | ○ | ○ | ○ | ○ |
| Irritable if meals are missed | ○ | ○ | ○ | ○ |
| Depend on coffee to keep going/get started | ○ | ○ | ○ | ○ |
| Get light-headed if meals are missed | ○ | ○ | ○ | ○ |
| Eating relieves fatigue | ○ | ○ | ○ | ○ |
| Feel shaky, jittery, or have tremors | ○ | ○ | ○ | ○ |
| Agitated, easily upset, nervous | ○ | ○ | ○ | ○ |
| Poor memory/forgetful | ○ | ○ | ○ | ○ |

| | | | | |
|---|---|---|---|---|
| Blurred vision | ○ | ○ | ○ | ○ |

| **Category 10 (High Blood Sugar/Hyperglycemia)** | **0** | **1** | **2** | **3** |
|---|---|---|---|---|
| Fatigue after meals | ○ | ○ | ○ | ○ |
| Crave sweets during the day | ○ | ○ | ○ | ○ |
| Eating sweets does not relieve cravings for sugar | ○ | ○ | ○ | ○ |
| Must have sweets after meals | ○ | ○ | ○ | ○ |
| Waist girth is equal or larger than hip girth | ○ | ○ | ○ | ○ |
| Frequent urination | ○ | ○ | ○ | ○ |
| Increased thirst and appetite | ○ | ○ | ○ | ○ |
| Difficulty losing weight | ○ | ○ | ○ | ○ |

| **Category 11 (Adrenal Fatigue or HPA Axis Dysregulation)** | **0** | **1** | **2** | **3** |
|---|---|---|---|---|
| Cannot stay asleep | ○ | ○ | ○ | ○ |
| Crave salt | ○ | ○ | ○ | ○ |
| Slow starter in the morning | ○ | ○ | ○ | ○ |
| Afternoon fatigue | ○ | ○ | ○ | ○ |
| Dizziness when standing up quickly | ○ | ○ | ○ | ○ |
| Afternoon headaches | ○ | ○ | ○ | ○ |
| Headaches with exertion or stress | ○ | ○ | ○ | ○ |
| Weak nails | ○ | ○ | ○ | ○ |

| **Category 12 (Hyper-functioning Adrenals or HPA Axis Dysregulation)** | **0** | **1** | **2** | **3** |
|---|---|---|---|---|
| Cannot fall asleep | ○ | ○ | ○ | ○ |
| Perspire easily | ○ | ○ | ○ | ○ |
| Under high amount of stress | ○ | ○ | ○ | ○ |
| Weight gain when under stress | ○ | ○ | ○ | ○ |
| Wake up tired even after six or more hours of sleep | ○ | ○ | ○ | ○ |

| | | | | |
|---|---|---|---|---|
| Excessive perspiration or perspiration with little or no activity | ○ | ○ | ○ | ○ |

| Category 13 (Mineral Deficiency & Kidney Function) | 0 | 1 | 2 | 3 |
|---|---|---|---|---|
| Edema and swelling in ankles and wrists | ○ | ○ | ○ | ○ |
| Muscle cramping | ○ | ○ | ○ | ○ |
| Poor muscle endurance | ○ | ○ | ○ | ○ |
| Frequent urination | ○ | ○ | ○ | ○ |
| Frequent thirst | ○ | ○ | ○ | ○ |
| Crave salt | ○ | ○ | ○ | ○ |
| Abnormal sweating from minimal activity | ○ | ○ | ○ | ○ |
| Alteration in bowel regularity | ○ | ○ | ○ | ○ |
| Inability to hold breath for long periods | ○ | ○ | ○ | ○ |
| Shallow, rapid breathing | ○ | ○ | ○ | ○ |

| Category 14 (Thyroid Hypofunction) | 0 | 1 | 2 | 3 |
|---|---|---|---|---|
| Tired/sluggish | ○ | ○ | ○ | ○ |
| Feel cold—hands, feet, all over | ○ | ○ | ○ | ○ |
| Require excessive amounts of sleep to function properly | ○ | ○ | ○ | ○ |
| Increase in weight even with low-calorie diet | ○ | ○ | ○ | ○ |
| Gain weight easily | ○ | ○ | ○ | ○ |
| Difficult, infrequent bowel movements | ○ | ○ | ○ | ○ |
| Depression/lack of motivation | ○ | ○ | ○ | ○ |
| Morning headaches that wear off as the day progresses | ○ | ○ | ○ | ○ |
| Outer third of eyebrow thins | ○ | ○ | ○ | ○ |
| Thinning of hair on scalp, face, or genitals, or excessive hair loss | ○ | ○ | ○ | ○ |

| | | | | |
|---|---|---|---|---|
| Dryness of skin and/or scalp | ○ | ○ | ○ | ○ |
| Mental sluggishness | ○ | ○ | ○ | ○ |

| Category 15 (Thyroid Hyperfunction) | 0 | 1 | 2 | 3 |
|---|---|---|---|---|
| Heart palpitations | ○ | ○ | ○ | ○ |
| Inward trembling | ○ | ○ | ○ | ○ |
| Increased pulse even at rest | ○ | ○ | ○ | ○ |
| Nervous and emotional | ○ | ○ | ○ | ○ |
| Insomnia | ○ | ○ | ○ | ○ |
| Night sweats | ○ | ○ | ○ | ○ |
| Difficulty gaining weight | ○ | ○ | ○ | ○ |

| Category 16 (Pituitary Hypofunction) | 0 | 1 | 2 | 3 |
|---|---|---|---|---|
| Diminished sex drive | ○ | ○ | ○ | ○ |
| Menstrual disorders or lack of menstruation | ○ | ○ | ○ | ○ |
| Increased ability to eat sugars without symptoms | ○ | ○ | ○ | ○ |
| Get dizzy standing up | ○ | ○ | ○ | ○ |

| Category 17 (Pituitary Hyperfunction) | 0 | 1 | 2 | 3 |
|---|---|---|---|---|
| Increased sex drive | ○ | ○ | ○ | ○ |
| Tolerance to sugars reduced | ○ | ○ | ○ | ○ |
| "Splitting"-type headaches | ○ | ○ | ○ | ○ |

| Category 18 (Males Only) | 0 | 1 | 2 | 3 |
|---|---|---|---|---|
| Urination difficulty or dribbling | ○ | ○ | ○ | ○ |
| Frequent urination | ○ | ○ | ○ | ○ |
| Pain inside of legs or heels | ○ | ○ | ○ | ○ |
| Feeling of incomplete bowel emptying | ○ | ○ | ○ | ○ |
| Leg twitching at night | ○ | ○ | ○ | ○ |

| Category 19 (Males Only) | 0 | 1 | 2 | 3 |
|---|---|---|---|---|
| Decreased libido | ○ | ○ | ○ | ○ |

| | | | | |
|---|---|---|---|---|
| Decreased number of spontaneous morning erections | ○ | ○ | ○ | ○ |
| Decreased fullness of erections | ○ | ○ | ○ | ○ |
| Difficulty maintaining morning erections | ○ | ○ | ○ | ○ |
| Spells of mental fatigue | ○ | ○ | ○ | ○ |
| Inability to concentrate | ○ | ○ | ○ | ○ |
| Episodes of depression | ○ | ○ | ○ | ○ |
| Muscle soreness | ○ | ○ | ○ | ○ |
| Decreased physical stamina | ○ | ○ | ○ | ○ |
| Unexplained weight gain | ○ | ○ | ○ | ○ |
| Increase in fat distribution around chest and hips | ○ | ○ | ○ | ○ |
| Sweating attacks | ○ | ○ | ○ | ○ |
| More emotional than in the past | ○ | ○ | ○ | ○ |

| **Category 20 (Menstruating Females Only)** | **0** | **1** | **2** | **3** |
|---|---|---|---|---|
| Perimenopausal | ○ Yes | | ○ No | |
| Alternating menstrual cycle lengths | ○ Yes | | ○ No | |
| Extended menstrual cycle (greater than 32 days) | ○ Yes | | ○ No | |
| Shortened menstrual cycle (less than 24 days) | ○ Yes | | ○ No | |
| Pain and cramping during periods | ○ | ○ | ○ | ○ |
| Scanty blood flow | ○ | ○ | ○ | ○ |
| Heavy blood flow | ○ | ○ | ○ | ○ |
| Breast pain and swelling during menses | ○ | ○ | ○ | ○ |
| Pelvic pain during menses | ○ | ○ | ○ | ○ |
| Irritable and depressed during menses | ○ | ○ | ○ | ○ |
| Acne | ○ | ○ | ○ | ○ |
| Facial hair growth | ○ | ○ | ○ | ○ |
| Hair loss/thinning | ○ | ○ | ○ | ○ |

| **Category 21 (Menopausal Females Only)** | **0** | **1** | **2** | **3** |
|---|---|---|---|---|
| How many years have you been menopausal? | | | | |

| Since menopause, do you ever have uterine bleeding? | ○ Yes | | ○ No | |
|---|---|---|---|---|
| Hot flashes | ○ | ○ | ○ | ○ |
| Mental fogginess | ○ | ○ | ○ | ○ |
| Disinterest in sex | ○ | ○ | ○ | ○ |
| Mood swings | ○ | ○ | ○ | ○ |
| Depression | ○ | ○ | ○ | ○ |
| Painful intercourse | ○ | ○ | ○ | ○ |
| Shrinking breasts | ○ | ○ | ○ | ○ |

| **Category 22 (Immunity)** | **0** | **1** | **2** | **3** |
|---|---|---|---|---|
| History of autoimmune disease | ○ Yes | | ○ No | |
| Family member(s) with autoimmune disease | ○ Yes | | ○ No | |
| Shortness of breath, trouble breathing, or wheezing | ○ | ○ | ○ | ○ |
| Cognitive issues such as headaches, brain fog, memory problems, difficulty concentrating, and mood swings | ○ | ○ | ○ | ○ |
| General fatigue and weakness | ○ | ○ | ○ | ○ |
| Muscle aches, joint pain, morning stiffness | ○ | ○ | ○ | ○ |
| Numbness and tingling | ○ | ○ | ○ | ○ |
| Light sensitivity, blurred vision, or red eyes | ○ | ○ | ○ | ○ |
| Temperature regulation problems | ○ | ○ | ○ | ○ |
| Numbness/tingling in extremities | ○ | ○ | ○ | ○ |
| Frequent sinus congestion/sinus problems | ○ | ○ | ○ | ○ |
| IBS or loose stools | ○ | ○ | ○ | ○ |
| Itchy, watery eyes | ○ | ○ | ○ | ○ |
| Skin: hives, flushing, itching | ○ | ○ | ○ | ○ |
| Multiple food sensitivities | ○ | ○ | ○ | ○ |
| Low blood pressure and/or rapid heart rate | ○ | ○ | ○ | ○ |
| Recent or history of frequent exposure to fumes, chemicals, or mold | ○ | ○ | ○ | ○ |

## *SCORING: GUT CHECK*

Review your answers and each section. The answers on the right-hand side (more threes and fours) indicate areas of higher priority. Every category has a tie to the gut, and some are bi-directional. For example, adrenal or stress imbalances can lead to gut issues and vice versa. Assess which categories have the highest ratings for you, and match your top categories to the five Gut Types to figure out your dominating gut type(s).

Category 1: Digestive Gut, Immune Gut
Category 2: Digestive Gut, Immune Gut, Toxic Gut
Category 3: Digestive Gut, Immune Gut, Toxic Gut
Category 4: Digestive Gut
Category 5: Digestive Gut, Immune Gut
Category 6: Digestive Gut, Immune Gut
Category 7: Digestive Gut, Toxic Gut
Category 8: Digestive Gut, Toxic Gut
Category 9: Digestive Gut, Hormonal & Metabolic Gut
Category 10: Digestive Gut, Hormonal & Metabolic Gut
Category 11: Hormonal & Metabolic Gut, Brain Gut
Category 12: Hormonal & Metabolic Gut, Brain Gut
Category 13: Toxic Gut, Hormonal & Metabolic Gut, Brain Gut
Category 14: Hormonal & Metabolic Gut
Category 15: Hormonal & Metabolic Gut
Category 16: Hormonal & Metabolic Gut
Category 17: Hormonal & Metabolic Gut
Category 18: Hormonal & Metabolic Gut, Brain Gut
Category 19: Hormonal & Metabolic Gut, Brain Gut
Category 20: Hormonal & Metabolic Gut, Brain Gut
Category 21: Hormonal & Metabolic Gut, Brain Gut
Category 22: Immune Gut, Toxic Gut

## *WHAT TO DO ABOUT IT*

Refer to the Resources: Eat & Supplement for Your Gut Type for specific insights about specific nutrition and supplements that may support you during the Total Gut Reset.

Also keep in mind: the more we continue to support the gut and address stress as a whole, the more likely it is that our symptoms will gradually subside.

# ASSESSMENT #2: THREE-DAY FOOD, MOOD, AND POO LOG

## *STEP 1: RATE YOUR HUNGER AND FEELINGS*

- Before the meal, rate your level of hunger/fullness on a scale of 1 to 10 with 1=starving, 5=neutral, and 10=stuffed.
- Note any feelings, thoughts, or updates you have before the meal. (For example, "I am craving sugar," "I am dragging," "I was eating on the go.")

## *STEP 2: LOG IT*

- Log what you ate. Some apps let you take a pic, too!

## *STEP 3: RATE YOUR FULLNESS & FEELINGS*

- After the meal, rate your level of hunger/fullness on a scale of 1 to 10 with 1=starving, 5=neutral, and 10=stuffed.
- Record any feelings or thoughts you have after the meal.

## *STEP 4: NOTE YOUR LIFESTYLE FACTORS*

At the end of each day, also record:

- When you moved your bowels, and what your poop looks like
- How much coffee/caffeine you drank that day
- How much water you drank that day
- Hours of sleep the night before
- Any exercise you did

Start with just three days. This log will help you understand how you currently think and feel daily, so you can begin a new mindfulness practice with food and your lifestyle that will help you figure out what may be driving positive or negative symptoms.

After your 3 day log, transition to the Gut Love Kickstart "Diet" to establish a baseline for an anti-inflammatory gut loving ecosystem—an excellent way to tune into your gut. (You can also find the guidelines in the back of this book).

## DAY 1 FOOD, MOOD, & POO LOG

| | What You Ate & Time | Supplements | Hunger Rating (1-10)* Before | Fullness Rating (1-10)* After | Mood/ Digestive Changes |
|---|---|---|---|---|---|
| Breakfast | | | | | |
| Snack (if any) | | | | | |
| Lunch | | | | | |
| Snack (if any) | | | | | |
| Dinner | | | | | |
| Snack/Post-Dinner (if any) | | | | | |

**1=famished, 5=neutral, 10=stuffed*

## LIFESTYLE REFLECTION

| | |
|---|---|
| Poo (Times & Texture) | |
| Caffeine Intake | |
| Water Intake | (designer; 8-10 glasses to check off) |
| Movement/Fitness & How You Felt | |
| Sleep (Hours Last Night) | |

## DAY 2 FOOD, MOOD, & POO LOG

| | What You Ate & Time | Supplements | Hunger Rating (1-10)* Before | Fullness Rating (1-10)* After | Mood/ Digestive Changes |
|---|---|---|---|---|---|
| Breakfast | | | | | |
| Snack (if any) | | | | | |
| Lunch | | | | | |
| Snack (if any) | | | | | |
| Dinner | | | | | |
| Snack/Post-Dinner (if any) | | | | | |

**1=famished, 5=neutral, 10=stuffed*

## LIFESTYLE REFLECTION

| | |
|---|---|
| Poo (Times & Texture) | |
| Caffeine Intake | |
| Water Intake | (designer; 8-10 glasses to check off) |
| Movement/Fitness & How You Felt | |
| Sleep (Hours Last Night) | |

## DAY 3 FOOD, MOOD, AND POO LOG

| | What You Ate & Time | Supplements | Hunger Rating (1-10)* Before | Fullness Rating (1-10)* After | Mood/ Digestive Changes |
|---|---|---|---|---|---|
| Breakfast | | | | | |
| Snack (if any) | | | | | |
| Lunch | | | | | |
| Snack (if any) | | | | | |
| Dinner | | | | | |
| Snack/Post-Dinner (if any) | | | | | |

**1=famished, 5=neutral, 10=stuffed*

## LIFESTYLE REFLECTION

| | |
|---|---|
| Poo (Times & Texture) *Use the Golden Poo Chart | |
| Caffeine Intake | |
| Water Intake | (designer; 8-10 glasses to check off) |
| Movement/Fitness & How You Felt | |
| Sleep (Hours Last Night) | |

# BONUS: FOOD INTOLERANCE & BLOOD SUGAR IMBALANCES

This assessment is divided into three many experiments to complete at your leisure.

## *EXPERIMENT #1: FOOD SWAP CHALLENGE*

Step 1. List your top five foods

Step 2. Replace your top five listed foods for three to seven days

Step 3. Observe how you feel using a three-day food log once more.

Step 4. Reintroduce your old favorite foods at the end

| The Top 5 Foods<br>I Eat (Most) Every Day | Replacement Foods |
|---|---|
| 1. | 1. |
| 2. | 2. |
| 3. | 3. |
| 4. | 4. |
| 5. | 5. |

# THREE TO SEVEN DAY FOOD LOG

*Note: For the most accurate assessment, seven days would be ideal.*

## DAY 1

| | What You Ate & Time | Supplements | Hunger Rating (1-10)* Before | Fullness Rating (1-10)* After | Mood/ Digestive Changes |
|---|---|---|---|---|---|
| Breakfast | | | | | |
| Snack (if any) | | | | | |
| Lunch | | | | | |
| Snack (if any) | | | | | |
| Dinner | | | | | |
| Snack/Post-Dinner (if any) | | | | | |

## DAY 2

| | What You Ate & Time | Supplements | Hunger Rating (1-10)* Before | Fullness Rating (1-10)* After | Mood/ Digestive Changes |
|---|---|---|---|---|---|
| Breakfast | | | | | |
| Snack (if any) | | | | | |
| Lunch | | | | | |
| Snack (if any) | | | | | |
| Dinner | | | | | |
| Snack/Post-Dinner (if any) | | | | | |

## DAY 3

| | What You Ate & Time | Supplements | Hunger Rating (1-10)* Before | Fullness Rating (1-10)* After | Mood/ Digestive Changes |
|---|---|---|---|---|---|
| Breakfast | | | | | |
| Snack (if any) | | | | | |
| Lunch | | | | | |
| Snack (if any) | | | | | |
| Dinner | | | | | |
| Snack/Post-Dinner (if any) | | | | | |

## *EXPERIMENT #2:* ***COCA'S PULSE TEST***

1. Pick the food you think is causing issues.
2. Take your resting heart rate for 60 seconds before putting the food in your mouth.
3. Chew the food for 30 seconds.
4. Take your resting heart rate again.
5. If your rate changes more than 6 beats per minute, it suggests a histamine or food sensitivity reaction.

## *EXPERIMENT #3:* ***DIGESTIVE SUPERPOWERS***

Observe how you feel with the following foods eaten alone:

- Complete protein source (chicken, beef, turkey)
  **What it may mean if you don't feel well:** low stomach acid

- Healthy fat (fish, fish oil, ghee, avocado, butter)
  **What it may mean if you don't feel well:** gallbladder congestion

- FODMAP foods (brussels sprouts, broccoli, cauliflower, onion, garlic)
  **What it may mean if you don't feel well:** Dysbiosis, SIBO, candida and/or poor gallbladder function

- Histamine-rich food (spinach, canned wild salmon or tuna, fermented foods)
  **What it may mean if you don't feel well:** Immune gut, metabolic endotoxemia

- Carb challenge (starchy tuber, like a sweet potato or butternut squash)
  What it may mean if you don't feel well: Dysbiosis, bacterial overgrowth and/or digestive enzyme deficiencies

## *EXPERIMENT #4:* BLOOD SUGAR CHECK IN

How do your blood sugar and gut bugs respond when you eat? To find out, take the following blood sugar assessment.

**Directions:**
Purchase a blood glucose meter to test your blood sugar over a period of three days (these do not need to be consecutive). Test and record your blood sugar during the following times:

1. First thing in the morning, after at least 12 hours of fasting, before breakfast
2. Just before lunch (no food between breakfast and lunch)
3. 45 minutes after you finish your last bite of lunch
4. 1 hour after that (no food in between)
5. 1 hour after that (no food in between)

**Interpretation:**
Ideal blood sugar levels, measured by blood work or a reliable glucose meter, should fall between 70-140 mg/dl. Levels will change during the day. The following are the range of normal readings throughout the testing times suggested above:

**Ideal Fasting Morning Glucose**

- 70-85 mg/dl

**During the Day**

- Before meals normal sugars are 70–99 mg/dl
- Post-meal sugars (taken two hours after meals) should be less than 140 mg/dl

**The following are the range for hyperglycemia (high blood sugar) readings:**

- While fasting, 130 mg/dl and higher (after not eating or drinking for at least 8 hours)
- Two hours after eating, higher than 180 mg/dl (note that people without diabetes rarely have blood sugar higher than 140 mg/dl after a meal, unless it's very large)

**The following are the measurements indicating hypoglycemia (low blood sugar):**

- While fasting, below 70 mg/dl (after not eating or drinking for at least 8 hours)
- One to two hours after eating, lower than 70 mg/dl (note that people with hypoglycemia may experience "reactive" hypoglycemia after eating—a drop, instead of rise, in blood sugar after eating)

# ASSESSMENT #3: THE GOLDEN POO CHALLENGE

**Directions**

What does your poo say about you? Take the Golden Poo Challenge.

Part 1: Keep a 3 day log of your daily poo patterns—when you go, what it looks like, and identify any "causes" of your poo. You can do this in conjunction with your Gut Check 3 Day Food, Mood & Poo Log (Assessment #2) and use the Golden Poo Chart as a guide.

Part 2: After you complete the log, evaluate it for areas to improve for the golden poo. If it's not golden, try 1 to 3 "golden poo hacks."

**Constipation**

- Use magnesium and/or buffered Vitamin C to "go" if you need support
- Chew your food until fully liquified and slow down
- Sea moss, 1-2 spoonfuls daily
- Probiotics: Lactobacilli plantarum
- Squatty Potty
- Sit up straight during the day (No slouching! Watch that posture.)
- Take a "pro-kinetic" in the morning and evening to stimulate bowels naturally
- Eat food w/ breakfast (can create 'bulk' in your stool to go #2)
- Sip Smooth Move Tea

- Move your body daily; but avoid 'chronic cardio' (can constipate your more)
- No laying down or intense exercise directly after eating
- Drink enough water + 1 serving minerals
- Avoid drinking out of plastic water bottles (causes gut inflammation)
- Add in a soluble fiber supplement (psyllium husk, pectin, flaxseed, partially hydrolyzed guar gum) and include soluble fiber, pickled veggies and resistant starch in diet (ie. cooked summer squash, sautéed greens, winter squash, roasted carrots, pickled beets, etc)
- Avoid raw veggies and raw salads
- Eat warm and room temp foods
- Possibly avoid high FODMAPs while supplementing w/ soluble fiber, probiotics and oil of oregano or berberine
- Love your gallbladder: digestive bitters with meals
- Coffee enemas
- Take Chlorella tablets
- Jump up and down in place (rebounding) if you feel "stuck"
- All 4's: table top position (hands and knees)
- Squeeze your colon acupuncture point (right hand inner web)
- Abdominal massage
- Hypnosis for digestion and meditation

**Loose Stools**

- Chew your food until fully liquified and slow down
- Best Probiotics: Lactobacillus rhamnosus GG, Saccharomyces boulardii, Bifidobacterium lactis, Lactobacillus casei & D-lactate free formulas
- Apple cider vinegar shots (Next level: Add 1 teaspoon of soda bicarbonate to a glass and pour 10 ml of hot water over it. Now add 1 teaspoon of ACV and 1 liter of mineral water to it)
- "Lemonade" (Mix the juice of 1 lemon with a glass of water + 1 tsp raw honey)

- Activated coconut charcoal https://amzn.to/3Jh5fp8 at bed w/ a big glass of water
- IB Guard capsules (peppermint oil)
- Black seed oil
- Short-term (7-14 days) antimicrobial herbs w/ meals (berberine, oregano, thyme, goldenseal, etc.)
- Fenugreek seeds (Mix a 1 tbsp coconut yogurt/plain yogurt or applesauce with fenugreek seeds)
- Yogurt, half cup (grassfed, coconut)
- Drink plenty of clear liquids, including water, broths and fresh vegetable juices
- Vanilla water: 1 tbsp pure vanilla + 6 ounces water + 1 tsp raw honey
- Sip chamomile or peppermint tea
- Fresh peppermint
- Avoid coffee, caffeine, artificial sweeteners, refined sugar, alcohol, gluten, soy and industrial seed oils (canola, vegetable, grapeseed, sunflower, safflower)
- Avoid raw fruits and veggies
- Carob powder (mix in applesauce, yogurt, smoothies, sweet potatoes; take with plenty of water)
- Ginger (Add grated ginger to a cup of water and boil it for 5 to 10 minutes. Strain and cool the water and drink a tablespoon after every hour)
- Cinnamon (add to drinks or food)
- Resistant starch: cooked and cooled white rice/potatoes/oats, green plantains/bananas, potato starch/plantain flour, cassava/arrowroot/coconut flour, lentils/beans
- Eat an apple a day (if not FODMAP sensitive)—contain pectin which is what helps diarrhea by hardening the stool
- Consider food intolerances: dairy, histamines, high FODMAPs, carbohydrate malabsorption
- Consider treating SIBO and candida

# ASSESSMENT #4: YOUR HEALTH STORY

**Directions**

Create a health Story Timeline for yourself, identifying at least five to 10 stressors, triggers, circumstances, or events that comprise your own health story, your journey. These can be mental, emotional, and physical factors. This timeline will help you piece together the factors which may have contributed to your health, as well as understand any current stressors continuing to drive your symptoms.

Some examples may include:

## *BIRTH HISTORY*

microbial dysbiosis triggers:

- C-section baby
- Formula fed
- Antibiotics before age two
- Processed foods as a kid

## *CHILDHOOD HISTORY*

- Antibiotics
- Processed foods
- Picky diet
- Chronic ear, sinus, or strep infections
- Trauma
- Broke my arm
- Bullied at school
- Didn't fit in/self-conscious
- Financial stress in my family
- Constantly people-pleasing
- Isolated/not a lot of friends

## *HEALTH AND LIFESTYLE HISTORY*

- Long-term medication use/birth control
- Surgeries
- Traumas
- Mold exposure
- Illness or infection
- Sleep deprivation
- Chronic conditions/diagnoses

- Addiction
- Parents divorced
- Lost my job
- Eating disorder began
- Depression
- Diagnosed with Hashimoto's

## *FOODS*

- Less than eight cups of water/day
- Low fat diet
- Eat gut-irritating foods (canola oil, restaurant meals frequently, refined grains)
- Consume artificial sweeteners
- Low fiber intake
- No variety
- Packaged and processed foods
- Over-eating
- Restrictive diets
- Binging or purging
- Coffee dependence
- Went keto
- Stopped eating meat

## *CURRENT HEALTH AND LIFESTYLE STRESSORS*

- Poor sleep
- Night Shift work
- Constipation
- Anxiety
- High work demands
- Sitting most of the day
- Netflix/TV binging
- Under-eating
- Overtraining or sedentary lifestyle
- Frequent sickness
- Moving stress
- Relationship stress
- Smoking
- Drinking most nights of the week
- Rely on coffee to function

### *GUT-BRAIN CONFLICTS*

- Was there a time where you heard something or saw something you could not "digest" but you had to, or when you were afraid for survival? (morsel conflict)
- Was there a time when someone was having a serious go at you and you had to protect yourself? (attack conflict)
- Was there a time when someone said something to you, even though you knew it was wrong and you let them get away with it but it devastated your self-esteem? or When you felt worthless or When your self-esteem was shattered? (self devaluation/esteem)
- Was there a time where you were left all alone to fend for yourself, you were abandoned?(territory)
- Was there a time when someone was trying to take something or someone away from you where you wanted to fight them or run away from them but could not? (territory/separation)

**You don't have to list EVERYTHING, but include at least five stressors from your past and five current stressors in your present to visually see what has potentially contributed to you not feeling your best or being where you want to be.*

## ASSESSMENT #5: CLINICAL LAB TESTS

When in doubt, the number one thing I consider when trying to determine if a certain test is the right option is this: will the results of the test change the treatment protocol?

The answer to that question helps to instantly rule out unnecessary testing. Generally, in terms of testing, *less* is more. Although there are tons of tests you *can* run that may be beneficial, I prefer to start as *lean* as possible and add additional testing if needed.

The tests you do need form a triple threat:

1. Functional blood chemistry panel (CBC, metabolic panel, lipid panel, iron panel, complete thyroid and hormone panel, Vitamin D)
2. Gut microbiome testing: comprehensive stool analysis
3. Optional wild card: specific to *you*
    - Hair or serum mineral analysis

- SIBO breath testing
- Saliva & urine hormone cortisol testing
- Gluten-intolerance and gluten cross-reactivity testing (bloodwork, Cyrex Array 3 and/or 4)
- Mold/mycotoxin testing (urine and blood work markers)

## *INSIDER TIP: DON'T GO IT ALONE.*

One of the most important steps for running lab tests and addressing findings appropriately is to work with a skilled practitioner who understands functional medicine.

Note: Not all practitioners are created equal. Don't assume that just because a clinician has letters behind their name or a white lab coat or that they "know all"; do your due diligence in asking questions, as well as looking for someone who does not promise you cures or claim to know it all. Also, look for someone with personal experience (either themselves or like patients) in "getting to the root cause(s)". Other notable qualities may include:

1. Not one-size-fits-all: Do they prescribe the same exact leaky gut plan or parasite cleanse for everyone they see? Or do they put a fresh pair of eyes on your case?
2. Someone who understands mechanisms vs. symptoms. IBS and bloating? What mechanism is driving the IBS and bloating? Gallbladder? SIBO from low stomach acid? Sleep deprivation?
3. Excessive lab testing and supplements. Functional labs should only be used if they will change the direction of treatment. Supplements should be explained (why are you taking them?), therapeutic (short term) and minimal as possible? (More than 5-8? Run).
4. Treat the person, not the diagnosis or test. Test positive for mold toxicity, but no signs or symptoms of mold illness? Maybe it was picked up from your food! You want a practitioner who treats you. Not just a lab marker.
5. Exit strategy. What's next after your Kickstart phase? How do you transition your diet if at all? What's your supplement schedule look like after 30 to 60 days?

# APPENDIX

| Organ | Conflict Content |
|---|---|
| Adrenal cortex | Moving- into- wrong- direction- conflict, or being thrown off the track. |
| Adrenal medulla | Unable to withstand- stress- conflict. |
| Anterior lobe of pituitary gland | Inability-to-get- chunk- conflict; i.e. the chunk is out of reach, or the child/family cannot be fed, because the individual is too tiny. |
| Bladder- sphincter | Territory- marking- conflict. |
| Bladder- submucosa | Ugly- conflict i.e. something felt as a mess, or something felt very ugly. |
| Bladder mucosa | Territory-marking- conflict; i.e. to define a limit or a position. |
| Blind gut - appendix | Ugly- indigestible- anger- conflict; e.g. often connected with ugly situations. |
| Blood vessels - arteries | Self-devaluation-disability-conflict; according to the corresponding localization. |
| Blood vessels- veins | Self-devaluation; according to the conflict content and the organ. |
| Bones | Inferiority-conflict; conflict contempt according to the skeletal parts: cervical spine- intellectual-moral- self devaluation conflict-shoulder/arm-partner-child-self devaluation-conflict; thoracic spine- central personality-self devaluation-conflict; femoral neck- cannot speak out something; pubic bone- sexual self-devaluation- conflict; knee- sport/flexibility; foot- flexibility-self devaluation-conflict; hand- unhandiness-self devaluation conflict. |
| Branchial arch ganglia | Fear- of- frontal- attack- conflict; something is coming right at us and we cannot protect ourselves from it, nor do anything. |

| | |
|---|---|
| Breast intraductal | Separation- fear- conflict; i.e. from mate, child, mother, home or nest. |
| Breasts mammary glands | Worry- argument or nest- conflict; i.e. mate, child, mother, home, nest |
| Bronchial asthma | Territory- fear- conflict; i.e. somebody is threatening to invade our territory, or wants to leave it without our permission. |
| Bronchial mucosa | Sensory territory- fear conflict. |
| Bronchial tubes goblet cells | Inability- to- salivate-air-chunk-conflict; i.e. the fear of suffocation, or the choke on something. |
| Cardiac smooth muscles | Peristaltic- transportation of blood. |
| Cardiac muscle myocardium | Being- overwhelmed- conflict. |
| Cartilage | Minor-self devaluation-conflict. |
| Colon | Ugly- indigestible- anger- conflict. |
| Connective tissue | Minor-self devaluation-conflict; different conflict contents according to the localization. |
| Coronary veins | Sensory territory- competition- fear- conflict |
| Esophagus | Inability- to- swallow-chunk- conflict; something that we want to incorporate, but suddenly we are not able to. |
| Eustachii tubes | Hearing conflict; i.e. cannot catch (believe) or get rid of an information chunk |
| Eye - cornea | Strong-visual- separation- conflict; i.e. we lost sight of somebody or something. |
| Eye - crystalline lens | Visual-separation- conflict; i.e. we lost sight of somebody or something. |
| Eye - Iris | Inability- to-catch-or- avoid-light-particles- conflict. |
| Eye - lacrimal glands | Visual-chunk-conflict; i.e. the inability to get rid of something that we did not see on time, the inability to catch (believe) something. |
| Eye - lacrimal glands ducts | To-be-seen-or-not-want-to-be-seen-conflict. |
| Eye - Retina | Separation- loss- conflict; i.e. we lose somebody, we separate or split from a loved person or lose sight of them. |
| Eye - Retina | Fear or rear attack conflict fear of something we cannot that is threatening or lurking from behind. |
| Eye- vitreous body | Fear-of-rear- attack- conflict; Somebody or something threatening us unexpectedly and frightening us. |
| Facial paralysis- facioplegia | To-loose-the-face-conflict; or the fear to be fooled. |

| | |
|---|---|
| Fatty tissue - adipose tissue | Minor- self devaluation- conflict; i.e. devaluation-conflict related to the part of the body that we feel unaesthetic, too skinny or too fat. |
| Gallbladder ducts | Territory-anger-conflict; i.e. violation of the limits to a neighbor, rival, mate, co-worker, etc., angry about somebody who invaded our territory. |
| Hair- alopecia | Separation conflict; depending on personal associations with certain parts of the body i.e. we used to caress the head of a loved one, and now we don't we do not anymore. |
| Hearing | Hearing- conflict; not wanting to hear something |
| Intestine- greater omentum | Ugly- abdomen- conflict. |
| Intestine- small | Indigestible-chunk-conflict; i.e. cannot digest something an indigestible anger is often an aspect of the starvation |
| Intestine- smooth muscles | Inability-to-move-chuck-conflict. |
| IKidney- parenchyma | Water- fluidity- conflict; i.e. somebody was almost drowned, or suffered a flooding |
| Larynx- asthma | Shocking-fear-conflict |
| Larynx mucosa | Shocking-fear or loss-of-speech -conflict; i.e. fear of an unexpected danger or to be paralyzed with fear, or not knowing what to say. |
| Liver parenchyma | Starvation- existence - conflict |
| Lungs - alveoli | Existence - and- fear- of- death- conflict; i.e. fear of death in accidents, analysis shock, etc. |
| Lymph nodes | Minor-self devaluation-conflict; conflict content according to the skeletal parts. |
| Lymph vessel | Minor- self devaluation-conflict; special disability of the localization according to the corresponding skeletal part. |
| Metab, thalamus | Self-renouncement- conflict; i.e. if I only was dead. |
| Middle ear | Hearing-conflict; i.e. cannot catch (believe) nor get rid of an information chunk. |
| Motorial paralysis (MS ) | Paralyzing conflict; i.e. cannot flee or come along (legs), cannot hold or repel arms, hands), cannot evade (shoulder and back muscles), to be at a loss. |
| Mouth | Inability- to- salivate to- get -chunk in or out conflict; i.e. cannot assimilate the food rightly. |
| Muscles - skeletal | Motion- self devaluation- conflict; i.e. cannot flee (legs), cannot repel or hold (arms ). |

| | |
|---|---|
| Nasal mucosa | Nose - stinking- conflict; i.e. being upset or angry about something something Is stinking or gets strongly on my nerves. |
| Navel | Excretory-conflict. |
| Oral cavity mucosa | Mouth- or- tongue- conflict; i.e. a conflict that has no to do with the mouth, the tongue or with savoring. |
| Ovaries | Profound- loss- conflict; i.e. child wife parents, friends' pet or ugly halfgenital conflict with a man. |
| Ovaries and testicles | Profound- loss- conflict; i.e. of a loved person, animal or object. |
| Palate | Inability- to - get-chunk-in-or-out-conflict; i.e. the inability to spit out something, or after getting something, the inability to swallow it. |
| Pancreas | Territory-anger or territory- fear-conflict; i.e. disputes and anger with neighbors, boss, partner or mate, etc. |
| Pancreas | Anger-fight-conflict; i.e. fight, anger, disputes about people, money, objects, heirship, or another "chunk". |
| Pancreas beta cells | Resistance-conflict; i.e. to resist or fight against somebody or something. |
| Pancreas mucosa | Territory-anger or identify conflict. |
| Pancreas alpha cells | Fear- disgust-conflict; i.e. to find somebody or something scary, disgusting. |
| Paranasal sinuses mucosa | Nose-stinking- conflict; i.e. something is stinking, or a conflict related to the smelling. |
| Parathyroid glands | Inability- to- get -chunk- in- or- out- conflict. |
| Parotid glands | Inability- to- salivate- to- get- chunk- in- or out- conflict. |
| Parotid glands, excretory ducts | Inability- to-eat- or- to-salivate-conflict. |
| Penis | The conflict of not being able to penetrate a narrow or dry vagina. |
| Pericardium | Attack- against- the heart conflict; i.e. a real attack or an associated attack against the heart. |
| Periosteum | Brutal- separation- conflict; i.e. is caused by a pain that we inflicted on somebody, or that we suffered ourselves. |
| Pharyngeal tonsil | Inability-to-let-off-or-swallow-chunk-conflict; i.e. cannot (accept) something (an assured residence or a job gets suddenly snapped up) |
| Pharynx- mouth | Inability- to- get- chunk- conflict. |
| Pleura | Attack against the chest conflict; i.e. a real or not attack against the chest |

| | |
|---|---|
| Prostate | Ugly- territory-conflict; i.e. The younger girlfriend abandons an elderly man in favor of a younger man. |
| Rectum - Sigma | Ugly- excretory- conflict. |
| Rectum submucosa | Ugly- excretory- conflict. |
| Rectum mucosa | Female- identity- conflict; i.e. is not knowing where she belongs to, or where to go, or the inability to take a decision. |
| Rectum muscles | Inability to mark the territory sufficiently. |
| Renal pelvis mucosa | Territory- marking- conflict; i.e. the inability to limit or mark the territory from inside (similar to the identity conflict) i.e. not knowing what to do or which view to subscribe to. |
| Skin dermis | Defilement- deformed- identity- trauma -conflict; i.e. feeling deformed or scarred. |
| Skin-dermis, neurofibroma | Contact- conflict; the opposite of the separation conflict; on the same organs respectively. |
| Skin epidermis, outer dermis | Separation- conflict; i.e. the loss of physical contact or the loss of the contact to the mother, the flock, the family, or friends. |
| Skin vitiligo | Brutal- ugly- separation conflict; i.e. from a loved or idolized person. |
| Smell | Smelling conflict; not one thing to stand something. |
| Spermatocyst | Sensory territory- competition- fear- conflict; the same conflict constellation as on coronary veins. |
| Spleen | Blood loss - self devaluation-conflict |
| Stomach-duodenum | Anger-digestion-conflict; i.e. the inability to digest a situation, like anger with relatives, coworkers or friends. |
| Stomach - esophagus mocusa | Inability-to-swallow-chunk-conflict; i.e. cannot swallow (accept) something on the impulse to spit it out again |
| Stomach - large curvature | Inability-to-digest-chunk-conflict; something lies in the stomach, mostly related to job, family, money, property, relationships, legal issues etc. |
| Sublingual glands excretory ducts | Inability-to-eat-or-to-salivate-conflict. |
| Sublingual salivary glands | Inability-to-get/salivate/get-out-chunk-conflict |
| Teeth bones | Bite-conflict; i.e. self-devaluation of not-allowed-to-bite, or somebody who would like to bite or to strike, but is not allowed or does not have the heart to do it. |

| | |
|---|---|
| Teeth enamel | Defensive, not-allowed-to-bite-conflict; contents, with the different evolutionary conflict contents, according to the teeth: incisor = not-grabbing, canines = not-catching, molars/grinders = not-grinding. |
| Tendons | Minor-self devaluation-conflict. |
| Testicles | Profound-loss-conflict; i.e. to lose a person, pet or object, or a ugly half genital |
| Thyroid - excretory ducts | Powerless conflict |
| Thyroid glands | Inability-to-get-chunk-in-or-out conflict, i.e. cannot get or get rid of something. |
| Ureter mucosa | Territory-limit/marking-conflict; i.e. the inability to limit the territory from the inside, or to mark the limits of the territory |
| Urethral mucosa | Territory-limit/marking-conflict; i.e. the inability to limit the territory from inside, or to mark the limits of the territory. |
| Uterine tube | Ugly-half genital-conflict with a male person. |
| Uterus | Ugly-half genital-loss-conflict. |
| Uterus - mouth and neck | Loss-of-territory/fear-conflict; The conflict content is analogue to the coronary veins (Coronary veins ulcer); depending on the handedness, hormonal situation and conflict content. |
| Uterus muscle | Self-devaluation of not-getting-pregnant-conflict. |
| Uterus neck muscle | Self-devaluation-conflict; i.e. cannot hold the pregnancy or the penis. |
| Vagina | Bartholini glands |
| Vaginal-dryness | conflict; i.e. cannot produce enough vaginal mucus for the coitus. |
| Vagina mucosa | Not-being-copulated-conflict; i.e. cannot or is not allowed to complete the copulation. |

# AUTHOR BIO

Dr. Lauryn is a former TV news journalist gone "health detective" and gut love + food freedom expert who helps clients worldwide to get to the root cause of their greatest health challenges and optimize how they look, move, feel and think.

As a Doctor of Occupational Therapy, Clinical Nutritionist and Functional Medicine Practitioner, Dr. Lauryn's work is inspired by her over 25 years of clinical and personal experience spent overcoming 10 chronic health issues diets, doctors and Dr. Google could not solve. Today, as a specialist in Gut Health, Non-Toxic Living and a Non-Diet Approach to Healing, she's made it her life mission to help others turn their greatest setbacks into their greatest comebacks.

Made in the USA
Columbia, SC
18 January 2024

30622591R00165